PATHFINDERS OF THE HEART

PATHFINDERS OF THE HEART

The History of Cardiology at the Cleveland Clinic

WILLIAM C. SHELDON, M.D.

To order additional copies of this book, contact:
Xlibris Corporation
1-888-795-4274
www.Xlibris.com
Orders@Xlibris.com
48613

CONTENTS

DEDICATION

This effort is dedicated to our forbearers who pioneered this great adventure.

It is also dedicated to Marge, Scott and John, and to the memories of Mark and David, whose love and sacrifice allowed me to have the incredible experience of the past forty-seven years.

WCS

PREFACE

Seventy-five years ago, in the midst of the Great Depression, the Cleveland Clinic launched a new department, *Cardiorespiratory Disease*. With the refinement of specialties in American medicine it became known as the *Department of Cardiology*. This is a story about its people. Leaders with imagination and wisdom who created an extraordinary enterprise in cardiology and a unique partnership with cardiac surgery that succeeded despite the challenges and conflicts. It is also the story of the workers who shouldered the burden, and the organization that provided the supportive environment.

Although the work of Cardiac Surgery and Cardiology has been intimately intertwined over the years, and the success of the cardiovascular effort at the Cleveland Clinic could not have occurred without this partnership, this story is told from the perspective of Cardiology and, regrettably, inclusion of all the staff and accomplishments of Cardiac Surgery are beyond the scope of this book. In addition, people and events in Cardiology at Cleveland Clinic Florida also could not be included.

I am greatly indebted to Dr. William L. Proudfit and Dr. Earl K. Shirey for their advice and many valuable contributions. They were there when many of these events happened and I was not. Their reminiscences are important. Also I extend my gratitude to Eric Topol, Steve Ellis, Brian Griffin, Mike Lincoff, Steve Nissen, Pat Tchou, Jim Thomas and Jim Young who helped me fill in some of the details for the chapter on The Topol Years and hope that I have represented them fairly. I am also indebted to Dr. J. Willis Hurst for his willingness to review the manuscript and contribute a Foreward. Carol Tomer and Fred Lautzenheiser of the Cleveland Clinic Archives Office have been extremely helpful in providing illustrations and background information; to both, my sincere thanks.

When I was younger I could remember everything, whether it happened or not; but my faculties are decaying now and soon I shall be so that I cannot remember any but the things that never happened.

Mark Twain

FOREWARD

I jumped at the chance to read *A History of Cardiology at the Cleveland Clinic*. Bill Sheldon had asked me to write a short Foreword to accompany the manuscript he had written. So I was able to savor the behind-the-scenes tales of the many people I knew who were responsible for development of Cardiology and Cardiac Surgery at the Cleveland Clinic. It is all there, at times with the bark off.

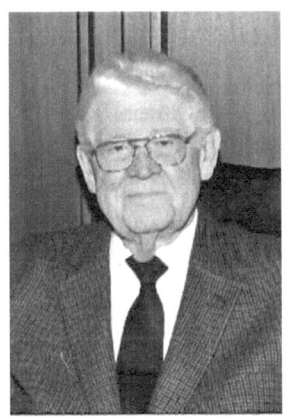

Sheldon's well-written and carefully-documented treatise is a gem of a book. He reports the entertaining stories of the chiefs and Indians that make the place successful and interesting. Sheldon asked me to write the piece because I, Professor and Chairman Emeritus, Department of Medicine, Emory University, Atlanta, Georgia, am old enough to have known the people involved from the beginning of the story and have witnessed the development for over 50 years.

J. Willis Hurst M.D.

I knew Carlton Ernstene who started it all at the embryonic Cleveland Clinic. There were only a few cardiologists in the country in the forties of the previous century. He was one of them. He had trained with Sam Levine. He was a calm and solid thinker who projected competence and knowledge. These attributes not only helped him create Cardiology at the Cleveland Clinic but helped develop cardiology in the country at large.

I knew William Proudfit best of all. He and I saw eye-to-eye on the value of coronary bypass surgery. I was initially skeptical but when the first clinical trial proved its value, I supported its development as strongly as I could. So when a scientific paper appeared in a journal, Proudfit and I would occasionally discuss it on the telephone. We talked many times and I appreciated his dry wit. Sheldon describes him perfectly.

I enjoyed Mason Sones. He was a brilliant worker whose prepared mind captured the moment when he accidentally injected contrast material into the coronary artery of a patient. When nothing serious happened to that patient, he recognized the enormous value of the procedure—giving birth to coronary arteriography. This, of course, changed the approach to the diagnosis and treatment of coronary disease. I enjoyed the man because you never knew what he would say or do. Sheldon's description of him is priceless.

I was privileged to know Rene Favaloro, the genius from Argentina. His early preparatory work at the Cleveland Clinic reveals why he became a leading surgeon in coronary bypass surgery. Although he was not the first to perform coronary bypass surgery, he was the most influential major player in its development and usage. After enormous success in this country he felt drawn to his homeland and returned to Argentina. He developed a great institute there and brought superb cardiac surgery to his country. My visit to observe his accomplishments was one of the highlights of my career. I received perhaps one of his last letters. He wrote to tell me that his institute and his work were collapsing. He asked me to see if Ted Turner might help since Turner owned much land in Argentina. The letter was a signal of his acute depression over a turn of events that he could not control. Over that weekend I framed a response in my mind planning to tell him that I did not know Ted Turner but that I did know Tom Johnson at CNN and would talk to him—hoping that he could urge Ted Turner to help. Before I could dictate and mail my letter to Rene, the headline appeared—Favaloro was dead. I was shocked and saddened—I really liked that man and what he had accomplished in his life. Sheldon reports his accomplishments and credits him appropriately.

William Sheldon led the development of Cardiology at the Cleveland Clinic from 1975 to 1991. He was a highly skilled clinician and superb organizer. He was able to pull together the large group of people who make up Cardiology at the Cleveland Clinic. The place thrived and became increasingly well-known in cardiac surgery, hypertension, pediatric cardiology, and peripheral vascular disease.

Eric Topol led the group from 1991-2006. I knew Topol only from his writing and from his one visit to Emory University. He appears to be a creative and talented person.

Passages from this book by Sheldon will be quoted by the scholars of the future because they tell an important and entertaining story about cardiology and cardiac surgery in this country.

J. Willis Hurst, M.D.
Professor and Chair,
Department of Medicine Emeritus
Emory University School of Medicine
December 11, 2007

THE ERNSTENE YEARS
1932-1965

Arthur Carlton Ernstene was born in Parker, South Dakota in 1901. After graduating from high school in Nebraska City, Nebraska he attended the State University of Iowa, graduating in 1922, and then the State University of Iowa College of Medicine, graduating with an M.D. degree in 1925.

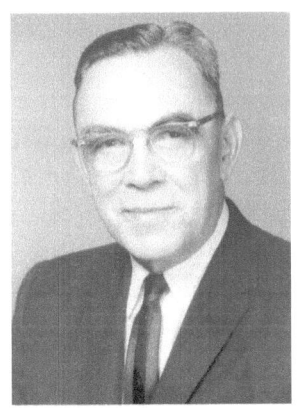

He was an intern at Henry Ford Hospital in Detroit in 1925-26 after which he moved to Boston as an assistant resident in Boston City Hospital's Thorndike Memorial Laboratory in 1926-27. He became an Assistant in Medicine at Harvard Medical School from 1927-30, an Instructor in Medicine in 1930-31, and a Faculty Instructor in Medicine in 1931-32.

A.C. Ernstene

During this time he served also as a resident physician in the Thorndike Laboratory in 1927-28 where he met Dr. Samuel A. Levine, and he began to study the erythrocytic sedimentation rate, noting that it was influenced by the hematocrit, leading to his description of a method to correct the erythrocytic sedimentation rate.[1] With Dr. Levine he studied electrocardiographic technics and, with the electrocardiograph, the effect of epinephrine in patients with angina pectoris. They had noted that arterial pressure became elevated during angina, but not with pain from other causes.

Beth Israel Hospital was a new hospital some distance away from the Thorndike Laboratory, but near Harvard Medical School. Dr. Herman Blumgart invited Dr. Ernstene to join him at Beth Israel as a research

Associate and assistant to Blumgart in his clinical practice in cardiology from 1929-32. Blumgart was an excellent clinician and a favorite of Harvard medical students. He was a great observer of cardiac physiology. He noted a relationship between increased venous pressure and orthopnoea, which he and Ernstene wrote about in 1930. Blumgart was one of the first cardiologists in American medicine, and later became the first editor of *Circulation.* Although he enjoyed his clinical practice, he was drawn to research, teaching, and writing. Ernstene became a devoted admirer and friend for life. He was invited to remain on the Harvard faculty and was promised a promotion.

While in Boston, Ernstene married Beatrice McGarvey, a proofreader who worked for a local publisher. They had one son, Marshall Paul, born in Boston March 24, 1930.

In 1932, Dr. Russell L. Haden, Chief of Medicine at the Cleveland Clinic and a hematologist with an interest also in rheumatic diseases, approached Dr. Ernstene about coming to the Clinic to organize a department of cardiorespiratory disease. Dr. Haden had started at the Clinic in September 1930, the year following the infamous fire of May 15, 1929, a disaster that had killed 123, including one of the founders, John Phillips[2] (Haden was his replacement). This was followed by the Great Depression that began in October 1929.

These were turbulent times in Boston, not only economically, but Beth Israel was experiencing internal political struggles. Ernstene's enthusiasm for the Harvard appointment was waning. Ernstene undoubtedly welcomed the opportunity to start a new department in a promising institution. He left Boston and was appointed head of the fourth specialty department at the Clinic's Division of Medicine, Cardiorespiratory Disease, in September 1932. (Diabetes and the Clinical Laboratories were established in 1921, Dermatology in 1923, and Endocrinology in 1929). In October, 1932 the medical staff and nonprofessional employees of the Clinic agreed to a ten percent cut in pay to help repay the heavy costs of the disaster and the cost of the new clinic building. There were additional pay cuts in 1933 as the Cleveland banks failed. Although research had been one of the three pillars in the mission of the Clinic, clinical practice assumed primary importance to maintain a revenue stream, and Ernstene was never able to return to original research.[3,4]

The Roots of Cardiology in the Post Disaster Era

When Ernstene arrived in 1932 [1]* the Clinic complex consisted of the reconstructed five story Clinic building, the site of the 1929 fire, an adjacent new three story clinic building completed in 1931, an eight story Research Building completed in 1928, a 275 bed Hospital building that extended from E 93rd St. to E 89th St. (the east extension was completed in 1929), and a power plant with laundry and refrigeration facilities.[2]

From 1932 to 1942 Ernstene developed a busy practice, and the Clinic slowly emerged from its economic doldrums. During this decade he published 66 papers on a variety of topics. He was certified in Internal Medicine in 1937, the first year after the Board was established. After Pearl Harbor and the outbreak of World War II the Clinic's U.S. Naval Reserve Medical Corps unit was called and he began active duty on March 1, 1942 as a Lieutenant Commander, with many other Cleveland Clinic staff members. He served as Chief of Medicine at a U.S. Naval Mobile Hospital in Auckland, New Zealand, and later at the U.S. Naval Base Hospital in Espiritu, New Hebrides.

The Clinic had been managed by a Board of Trustees that included its Founders, with George W. Crile as President until 1940 when failing vision necessitated his relinquishing the presidency to his industrialist/banker brother in law Henry Sherman.[3] The Board of Trustees was responsible for properties and finance, and a Medical Administrative Board was responsible for professional issues, Crile died in 1943 leaving William Lower the only surviving founder. After Crile's death Edward C. Daoust assumed the full-time Presidency of the Clinic and

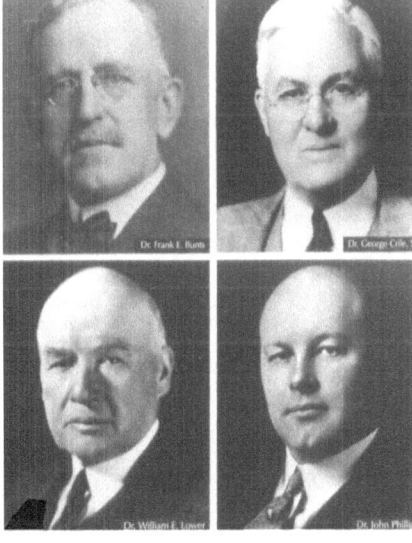

The Founders

Bunts	Crile
Lower	Phillips

---

* In this book endnotes are numbered in brackets [] and references are designated as superscripts, both appearing after each chapter.

3

became its chief administrative officer, reporting to the new Executive Committee of the Board and Sherman became the Chairman of the Board. A new Administrative Board of physicians represented the professional staff.

When Ernstene and his colleagues returned to their practices in 1944 and 1945 the Clinic again began to grow and prosper. An additional seven stories were added to the newer Clinic building in 1945.[3] Ernstene's department ultimately occupied one half of the eighth floor—Desk 81. An addition to the hospital building connected it with the research building. As the Clinic's governance organization developed Ernstene was appointed to several committees, first the committees on Professional Relations, Professional Policy, and Admissions in 1947, later the Personnel, Medical Practice, and Research committees in 1949. Specialty training in cardiology began in 1939 and Ernstene's first fellow was Jack Kinell.[4] [2]

Dr. H.S. VanOrdstrand became the second member of the Department of Cardiorespiratory Disease in 1939 as head of the section of Pulmonary Disease; this became a separate department in 1958.[3,5]

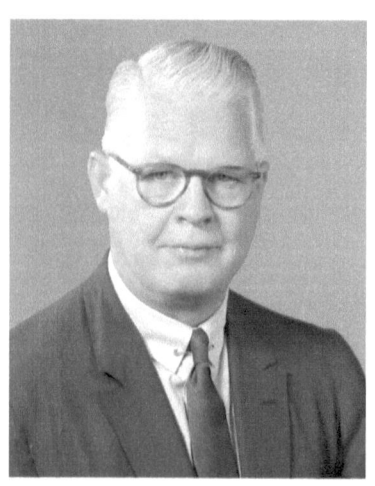

Fay A. LeFevre

Dr. Fay A. LeFevre became the third member of the Department of Cardiorespiratory Disease in 1942. He had been a Fellow in Medicine from 1932-34 after which he did postgraduate work in London, England at the National Neurological Hospital and the University of London with Sir Thomas Lewis and Sir George Pickering, and at the National Heart Hospital with Dr. Evan Bedford. On returning to Cleveland he entered private practice. When he joined the Clinic he was interested in peripheral vascular disease and in 1952 became head of a section of Peripheral Vascular Disease in the Department.

William L Proudfit, born in Connellsville, Pennsylvania in 1914, was a graduate of Harvard Medical School. He came to the Clinic as a fellow in Internal Medicine in 1940 and shortly thereafter he married Thelma

Janaske. When Dr. Jack Kinell completed a special fellowship in Ernstene's Department in 1941 Ernstene invited Proudfit to replace him the following year. Completing his fellowship in 1943, he received a commission in the U.S. Army Air Force. Proudfit was lean, with a somber appearance, but had a wonderful sense of humor. He dressed conservatively, and wore a short white coat following Ernstene's example. He befriended all. His humorous anecdotes were always studded with "hmm's" as if to anticipate the punch-line. After the war, on Ernstene's recommendation, Haden arranged for his appointment as a Staff

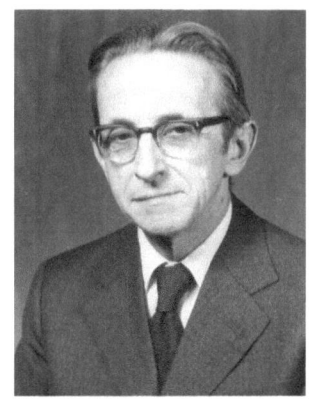

William L. Proudfit

Assistant (in Cardiorespiratory Disease). But a friend had told Proudfit about Dr. Frank N. Wilson at the University of Michigan and his interest in electrocardiography. Proudfit asked Ernstene for a letter of recommendation and after he was discharged from the Service in 1946 before he returned to Cleveland as a full staff member, he spent six weeks with Wilson in Ann Arbor learning electrocardiography—five days a week, eight hours a day. Wilson was not very interested in clinical medicine, but had several house officers who saw to his practice; Wilson supervised these fellows, while Proudfit observed.[6] [3]

John F. Whitman was a Fellow in Internal Medicine at the Clinic from 1946-1949. After two years at the assistant staff level he was appointed to the full Staff in Cardiorespiratory Disease in 1951. His tenure was short however; he had obstructive pulmonary disease and retired in 1960 on disability, and died six months later at age 42 from complications of pulmonary hypertension.

Richard N. Westcott, a graduate of Harvard Medical School, completed his residency in Internal Medicine at Cincinnati General Hospital in 1949 and a NIH postdoctoral research fellowship in the cardiac laboratory of Cincinnati General Hospital in 1951. Ernstene wanted Westcott because of his interest in clinical research. He was appointed to the Staff in the Department of Cardiorespiratory Disease in July 1951. He was an affable man but quickly realized that Ernstene could not provide him with the support, attitudinal as well as financial, that was necessary for a successful clinical research program. An excellent cardiologist, he shared the interpretation of electrocardiograms with

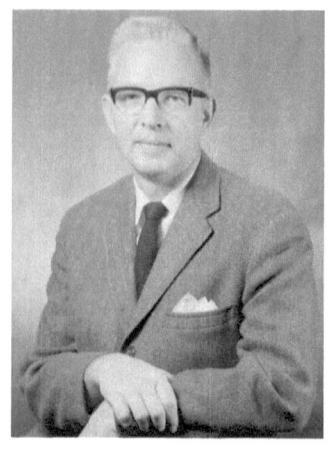

Richard N. Westcott

Proudfit and succeeded Proudfit as Director of the Electrocardiography Laboratory in 1966. In the early years he also worked with Van Ordstrand assisting with pulmonary function testing. Westcott had a busy practice and active career that was cut short in 1973 when at age 54 he died of lung cancer. [4]

Although the Clinic was to become known for its development of specialty practices, no one had the luxury of limiting himself to subspecialty interests, nor were subspecialties well developed nationally. The members of the Department of Cardiorespiratory Disease in the 1940's saw and cared for many patients with or without cardiorespiratory problems. Indeed, Ernstene's practice came to include many of Cleveland's community leaders—bankers, industrialists, and politicians. Proudfit looked after these patients as well, as Ernstene became more involved with national medical organizations. Proudfit was appointed to the Permanent Staff in November 1946.

Although Dr. Samuel A. Levine was a close friend of Dr. Frank Wilson, neither he nor Ernstene understood Wilson's theoretical ECG studies and their practical application. After Proudfit returned from Wilson's laboratory Ernstene recognized that he had superior knowledge in this narrow field and gave him total authority for the Electrocardiography Laboratory. He also immediately approved a modification of the electrocardiograph machines to record Wilson's central terminal leads. The Clinic was probably the first large institution after the University of Michigan to adopt this relatively new technique.

Ernstene, or "The Ace"—as his fellows referred to him privately (for his initials Arthur Carleton Ernstene), was known for his organization and punctuality. When he lived at the Park Lane Villa, a few blocks East and just North of Chester Avenue (when Euclid Avenue was still a rather fashionable part of Cleveland), he walked to work and would emerge from the elevator at Desk 81 at precisely 7:30 am. Hospital rounds started at precisely 8:00 and lasted for one hour. His day was filled with patients and consultations.

He had lunch alone in his office most days. Often after lunch he would close his door and nap for 10-15 minutes on his examination table, not to be disturbed. Only an important meeting would allow him to depart from his schedule. He spent little time socializing. The last hour of each day was for dictating reports on the day's patients. Reports completed, he departed at precisely 6:00 pm.

Proudfit later captured the essence of Ernstene's personality:[4]

> My office was next to Ernstene's for more than 20 years and slowly I learned something about him, but I never *knew* him. He had many friends but no intimates. He was handsome, personable, and short in stature. He did not exhibit the abrasiveness sometimes attributed to short men. Carl dressed conservatively in ready-made clothes, rarely of really current fashion. At work he wore a short white coat rather than the usual long one. He was always careful about expenditures, either personal or Clinic, but he was generous with friends. For the last 25 years of his life, he did not own an automobile and relied on public transportation. Carl had a quick, sincere smile and was capable of relaxed chatter but did not encourage it. His emotions were always controlled. He was quiet by nature and modest in demeanor. I had known him for more than 25 years before I knew that he had one brother, who was killed in a hunting accident. Carl was proud of having spent years in Boston at two hospitals and Harvard Medical School, but rarely mentioned it. He spoke well informally and in lectures and was never vulgar or profane. How he became president of so many medical societies I do not know because he was completely apolitical.
>
> Two characteristics of Ernstene impressed all observers: organization and efficiency. Dictation of letters and reports is a chore to most physicians but Carl never complained. Before leaving work each evening, he had dictated all letters, so his desk was clean in the morning. His letters were complete and easily understood. He dictated rapidly in a loud, clear voice and seldom made corrections. If one interrupted him during dictation, he stopped instantly and directed his attention to the visitor. At the end of the conversation,

Carl resumed his dictation, even in the middle of a sentence and before the visitor had reached the door. Letters of inquiry about former trainees were answered honestly but not bluntly. Once I heard him respond to such a letter about a former trainee who was not an Ernstene favorite. The entire response was "Dr. ___ spent the years ___ to___ with us and I knew him well."

If Carl planned to be away from the Clinic for more than a day or so he would ask me to care for his hospital patients. Once he was to vacation in Europe and he had not made a diagnosis in the case of an old man. Carl said jokingly that I should cable him if I made a diagnosis. The next morning on rounds the old fellow was almost unresponsive. I grasped an arm to help him sit for part of the examination—he screamed with pain and it was evident that his shoulders were almost immobile. The residents said that this was the first emotional response they had observed. The shoulder involvement is a relatively rare sign of hyperthyroidism; it was apparent that he had other signs also and a diagnosis of apathetic hyperthyroidism was made. I cabled Carl, "Hyperthyroidism" that day. Ernstene was an expert in the diagnosis of toxic thyroid. On returning to the Clinic and before shaking my hand he laughed and said, "I knew you were right." Even a blind hog finds an acorn once in awhile.

Carl was an outstanding physician. His idols were Francis Peabody and Herman Blumgart of Boston, both of whom treated patients rather than diseases. Early in his career at the Clinic he saw numerous patients daily because of the economic pressures created by the Great Depression, but after he returned from Naval service he cut down to six new patients daily, even when he was burdened by administrative duties and offices in national societies. These patients were examined by a resident but Carl repeated much of the history and physical examination. His hospital rounds started at exactly 8:00 a.m. and lasted one hour. After rounds, he carried out brief administrative duties and returned to his office. His resident was expected to have his first patient ready for him. Carl's notes were always concise, informative and neat. Treatment was simple and used as few drugs as possible.

In all phases of his clinical work, logic and experience dominated. He seemed to have a mental image of many diseases catalogued for instant extraction. One examinee for the American Board of Internal Medicine asked a Clinic trainee, "Who is this fellow Ernstene?" On receiving a cautious reply, the young man said, "He seems to have a computer for a brain. He flips through the database and finds the appropriate card that has all the answers. My problem was that I could not see the card." If Carl was asked to make an extemporaneous discussion at a conference, he opened with a few graceful comments and then "found the card" and delivered an excellent discussion.

Clinical medicine was a consuming passion for Carl. Most of his time in Boston was spent in research. First he developed the corrected erythrocyte sedimentation rate. Later, he did an extensive study of blood pressure response to pain. Over a period of several years, I had noted that hypertension accompanied anginal pain and occurred in the earliest stage of acute myocardial infarction. I mentioned this to Carl and he said that he had reported that while he was in Boston. I checked the Index Medicus and found the paper.[7] He found that non-coronary severe pain did not raise the blood pressure. So much for another of my "original" observations!

Referring to his dual responsibilities Proudfit commented:[4]

> He (Ernstene) said that I should be a "half-time" clinical cardiologist, seeing four new patients daily and three intra Clinic consultations as well as seeing former patients and making hospital rounds. I did not understand the arithmetic of "half-time" but I was happy to accept the offer.

David C. Humphrey joined the Department of Cardiorespiratory Disease in 1949 with a primary interest in hypertension. At that time most patients with hypertension were managed in the Division of Research under Drs. Irvine H. Page, A.C. Corcoran and Robert D. Taylor. In the 1940s it was beginning to be appreciated that hypertension had potentially serious ramifications, although there was little by way of treatment available. When it became apparent that hypertension was indeed a full fledged disease a separate Department of Hypertensive Disease was established in

1959 with Humphrey as its head.[3] Certain forms, malignant hypertension, renal hypertension, and hypertension associated with coarctation of the aorta were treatable: malignant hypertension was treated with sodium nitroprusside, coarctation was treated surgically.

During these years Page and colleagues continued to study and manage a special cadre of patients in the Research Division. Page, Harriet Dustan and Eugene Poutasse of the Department of Urology gained national fame for the Clinic with their contributions to the field of renal hypertension and the role of renal endarterectomy.[8] One of the early, live, national, closed-circuit television seminars was presented from the Clinic on this topic in 1959. Page and Bumpus discovered and synthesized angiotension in 1961.[9] Chlorthiazide was helpful in essential hypertension by reducing plasma volume. A new class of antihypertensive agents, alpha adrenergic blockers (guanethidine) was an important contribution.[10] In 1958 Page and Brown found that blood lipids could be lowered with dietary adjustments.[11]

Ernstene succeeded Haden as Chairman of the Division of Medicine in 1949. He was developing a national reputation. He was Secretary-Treasurer of the Cleveland Academy of Medicine in 1940-42, and a member of its Board of Directors in 1946-49. He was a founder and first President of the Cleveland Heart Society in 1949-51, and the Ohio State Heart Association in 1950-52. He was elected to the Association of American Physicians in 1949 [3].

In the American Heart Association he was Chairman of the Section on Clinical Cardiology in 1952-54, on the Executive Committee of the Board of Directors and Secretary of the Scientific Council in 1953, and President in 1960. He was certified by the American Board of Cardiovascular Disease and was a member of its Examining Board in 1956-61. He was on the Editorial Board of *Circulation* from 1958 until he retired. He was on the Executive Committee and Board of Governors of the American College of Physicians in 1958, a Regent in 1963-69, President in 1965-66, and elected a Master of the College in 1970.

Proudfit recalls another Ernstene vignette from the early 1950's:[6]

> Ernstene never missed a day of work after I returned in 1946.
> I recall only one occasion when he had a physical complaint

before his final illness. One Friday afternoon when he was about 50 years old he came into my office about 6:00 p.m. when he was sure that our corridor had been abandoned by others. He said, "Bill, listen to my heart." He had a pericardial friction rub and I said, "You have acute pericarditis." He replied, "Yes, that is what I thought." Then he admitted that he had pain all that day. His temperature was slightly elevated. I advised doing an electrocardiogram and reluctantly, he agreed. I did the recording, which showed changes typical of acute pericarditis. He secured the electrocardiogram and refused to have it placed in his record. I made notes about the visit but did not place them in his clinical record. I advised bed rest for a week but Ernstene said that was impossible. He made rounds on Saturday and Sunday and returned to full duty on Monday. He said that he had no pain on Monday. Whether he ever took the codeine that I prescribed, I do not know.

By 1950 surgical treatments were emerging for certain congenital heart diseases [12-17] and cardiac catheterization was being explored, not only for research in cardiac physiology, but also for diagnosis.[18,19] Ernstene decided that this was a new frontier in cardiology, and that the Clinic should have a cardiac catheterization laboratory. After looking at the emerging centers in congenital heart disease, he found a young fellow who was working in the laboratory of Dr. Robert Ziegler at the Henry Ford Hospital in Detroit.

The First Cardiac Catheterization Laboratory

F. Mason Sones Jr., born in Noxapater, Miss., had obtained his medical degree at the University of Maryland School of Medicine in 1943. He interned at the University of Maryland Hospital in 1944, and served in the U.S. Army Air Force from 1944 to 1946. He married Geraldine Newton in Baltimore on April 1 1945. After he was discharged from the Air Force he went to Henry Ford Hospital as a resident in internal medicine. While there he became intrigued with Dr. Ziegler's work with

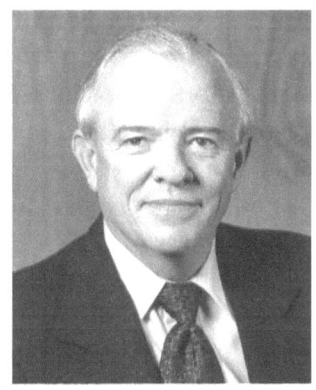

F. Mason Sones Jr.

cardiac catheterization in congenital heart disease, and went to work in his laboratory. In 1950 Ernstene invited him to come to Cleveland to establish a cardiac catheterization laboratory, primarily to conduct research, warning him, apologetically, that he doubted that cardiac cardiac catheterization would ever amount to anything as a useful clinical tool. Sones reluctantly accepted his somewhat muted invitation and began work in Cleveland October 1, 1950, as Director of the Cardiac Laboratory and Pediatric Cardiology in the Department of Cardiorespiratory Disease. He joined Ernstene, Proudfit and colleagues a Desk 81, and began to develop a catheterization laboratory on the third floor of the old clinic building that opened in 1952. Lucile Vanderwyst was its first head nurse.

Sones was short in stature, a feisty but gregarious fellow and a giant in intellect. Proudfit considered him a genius. He loved to talk and paid close attention in conversation. He was extremely energetic and intensely focused. Certain that cardiac catheterization would open new doors in cardiology, he enthusiastically set about to prove its value to Ernstene and all the disbelievers. He catheterized all the infants and children—and adults—with real or suspected congenital heart disease that were referred to him. It was not long before he had accumulated a substantial experience.

Robert Gross of Boston and Helen Taussig of Baltimore felt that infants under age two should not be catheterized since it was unlikely that they could survive any surgical treatment that might be available. When Sones found a surgically correctable problem, a patent ductus arteriosus or coarctation of the aorta, he recommended surgery even though some of these patients were severely ill. Fortunately the operative mortality was lower than expected. Although Gross and Taussig condemned this practice, Sones' experience was soon confirmed by others. Ernstene was pleased with this early success, and others learned that Sones' statements were the result of experience, not presumption. (The first Department of Pediatrics was established at the Clinic in 1951 with Dr. Robert Mercer as its head. An Obstetrics Department was initiated in 1955)

Cardiac Surgery Initiated

Donald B. Effler joined Dr. George Crile Jr., Dr. Tom Jones, Dr. Robert Dinsmore and Dr. Rupert Turnbull in the Division of Surgery, and was appointed Head of Thoracic Surgery in 1948. Effler had trained with Dr.

Brian Blades, a pioneer in thoracic surgery at the George Washington University in Washington. Effler was a tall handsome fellow, garrulous, with an arrogant demeanor and a cynical sense of humor. This estranged him from many colleagues, and most fellows were intimidated by him. [5] Effler focused more on thoracic surgery, at first for management of pulmonary tuberculosis, empyema, bronchiectasis etc, later for bronchogenic carcinoma. Not long after Sones arrived Effler began to perform operations for congenital heart disease. In addition to ligations of patent ductuses arterioses, resections of coarctations of the aorta, early operations included resections of vascular rings of the aorta, regarding which Effler and Sones wrote a paper in 1951.[20]

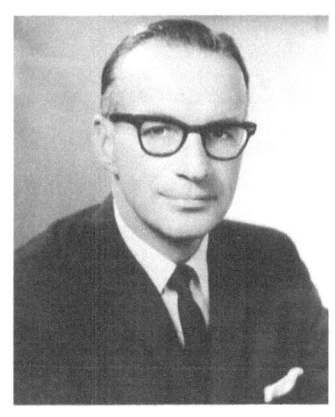

Donald B. Effler

Laurence Groves, a Harvard graduate, joined Effler in Thoracic and Cardiovascular Surgery in 1953. While Effler had the build of a basketball player, Groves looked more like a football player, with large hands. He became Effler's right hand man, as Shirey did later for Sones. He was modest and soft-spoken. In the operating room Effler was always talking, teaching, sometimes cajoling. Groves said little, but was a marvel of speed and efficiency. Favaloro recalls:

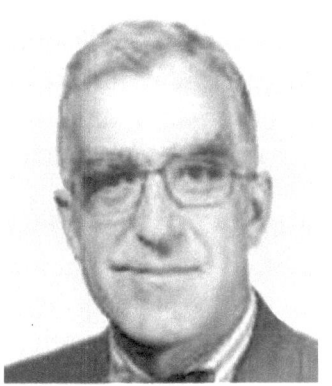

Laurence K. Groves

> He made even the most difficult maneuvers appear easy, thanks to his being ambidextrous. It was a real pleasure to watch him operate on small children, sometimes newborns, correcting congenital cardiac defects incompatible with life, or an esophago-tracheal fistula . . . . His main defect was his lack of communication, and he would remain silent even during the afternoon rounds when the whole team visited the patients. It was obvious that his relationship with Effler did not go beyond the strictly medical. In reality, he spoke very little, and when

he did, his English was difficult to understand, being devoid of emphasis. The Americans call this "mumbling."[21]

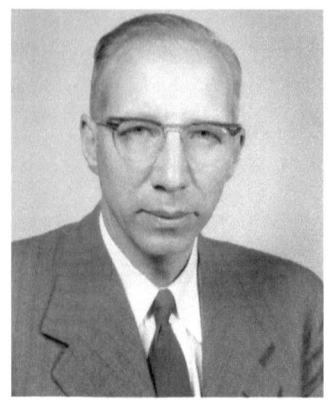

Willem J. Kolff

Willem J. Kolff arrived at the Clinic, also in 1950. He had trained at the University of Leiden, Netherlands, and later worked at the University of Groningen, and at Kampen where he experimented with cellophane tubes as a diffusing membrane in a process that would later become known as hemodialysis. He also observed that blood, dark when it entered the cellophane tube coil, became brighter as it exited having acquired oxygen from the atmosphere via the cellophane membrane, piquing his interest in blood oxygenators.[22]

Kolff formed a new Department of Artificial Organs in the Division of Research. Kolff and Irvine Page, the Chairman of the Division of Research, both strong minded individuals, were often in disagreement, leading to Kolff's transfer to the Division of Surgery. An ambitious innovator, Kolff developed hemodialysis for acute and chronic renal failure. [6] He also introduced one of the first methods for extracorporeal circulation, a disposable membrane type pump-oxygenator, and a method for achieving a controlled cardiac arrest in experimental animals, a cold potassium solution injected into the aorta. In 1954 Effler used both as he began to explore "open-heart" surgery.[23,24] Using Kolff's heart-lung machine and cold potassium cardiac arrest Effler performed the Clinic's first "open heart" surgery on a non-beating heart in February, 1956.[25][7] [8] Kolff became the third member of a triumvirate that laid the foundation for cardiac surgery at the Cleveland Clinic.

As cardiac surgery developed, the strong personalities of Kolff, Effler and Sones were perpetually in conflict, and soon they were at an impasse, which made communication impossible. Proudfit was appointed by the Board of Governors to chair daily 8:00 a.m. meetings of the three dissidents at which all communication was to be through Chairman Proudfit.[5, 26] As other types of extracorporeal circulatory devices replaced the membrane oxygenator Kolff devoted more time to perfecting hemodialysis. Later he developed one of the first prototypes for an implantable artificial heart. [9]

A rather problematic team that was beset with rivalry throughout their careers, Sones and Effler continued to build the joint cardiovascular effort that became the flagship of the Cleveland Clinic for the next generation.

Ernstene's first wife Beatrice died of complications of hypertension in 1952. During her final hospitalization Ernstene spent every waking hour with her. They had been married 23 years. Their son, Marshall, was named later by *Time Magazine* as one of the ten most brilliant young scientists in the United States.[6] Several years later Ernstene married Audrea Miller who had been a secretary at the Clinic.

Ernstene became increasingly busy with local and national responsibilities. He was a member of the Planning Committee that proposed the Board of Governors in 1955, as well as the first Board of Governors, from 1955-1957 and again from 1958-1963. A Clinic-wide reorganization in 1956 created Divisional committees[3] and the Medical Division Committee became Ernstene's sounding board.[5] He was a physician member of the Board of Trustees in 1961.

Largely on Ernstene's initiative, there was further evolution in the Division of Medicine. Dr. Victor DeWolfe had joined LeFevre's Section of Vascular Disease in 1952. Peripheral Vascular Disease was given full departmental status in 1955 with LeFevre as its Head. This was one of the few such departments in medical centers

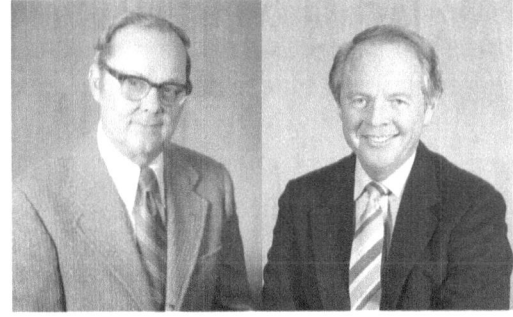

Victor DeWolfe   Jess R. Young

across the United States. (Dr. LeFevre also became Chairman of a newly established Board of Governors in 1955 and served in this capacity for thirteen years.[3,5]) Jess R. Young joined LeFevre and DeWolfe in Peripheral Vascular Disease in 1959. DeWolfe succeeded LeFevre as Department Chairman in 1961, and Young succeeded DeWolfe in 1976.

In 1956 Earl K. Shirey joined Sones as a special fellow. Born in Ligonier, Pennsylvania he attended Pharmacy School at the University of Pittsburgh and he married Mary Jean Broeseker in 1947 during his premedical training.

After a tour of duty in the U.S. Army, he attended Medical School at the University of Pittsburgh. He completed a residency in Internal Medicine at the Clinic in 1956. In the laboratory Shirey was a marked contrast to Sones. He appeared to be perfectly calm and perhaps he was. He spoke in a soft, compassionate voice to the patients and also to the laboratory personnel. Every motion was smooth and appeared unhurried. Quick to recognize his talent, Sones soon came to rely upon him in the clinic as well as in the hospital.

Royston Lewis, a convivial Welshman, was one of the early fellows in the cardiology training program that was funded by U.S. Public Health Service from 1958-62. On the morning of Roy Lewis' first day in the hospital, an infant was admitted on Sones' service. The heart rate was very rapid and an electrocardiogram showed atrial paroxysmal tachycardia. He was in severe congestive heart failure. Lewis went to Sones' office and reported his findings. Sones said, "Digitalize the hell out of him." He assumed that Lewis knew that he should give a mercurial diuretic also. Lewis was intimidated and feared to ask the dose of drugs to be given. Leaving Sones he decided to ask Shirey for help, because he had heard that Shirey was competent and kind. Shirey asked Lewis the weight of the infant and then gave him specific instructions about treatment. He was grateful to have Sones' philosophy translated into orders. That evening Sones saw the little boy after a busy day. By that time normal sinus rhythm had been restored and the boy was comfortable. Lewis learned something that day: when in doubt, find an expert.[6]

Later in the first year of his fellowship Lewis was witness to a landmark event as he assisted Sones in a catheterization during which the first injection of contrast medium into a coronary artery occurred and coronary arteriography became a reality (Chapter II). He was appointed to the staff in the Department of Clinical Cardiology in 1960.

In 1958 the Section of Pulmonary Disease was made a separate department with Van Ordstrand as its Chairman and the Department of Cardiorespiratory Disease then became the Department of Cardiovascular Disease.[3,5] In 1960 Sones' clinic and laboratory were given departmental status as the Department of Pediatric Cardiology and the Cardiac Laboratory. Ernstene's Department of Cardiovascular

Disease now became the Department of Clinical Cardiology (still located at Desk 81). Later, in 1967, with increasing attention to patients with valvular and coronary artery disease, The Department of Pediatric Cardiology was renamed the Department of Cardiovascular Disease and the Cardiac Laboratory

Ernstene continued as head of the Department of Cardiovascular Disease (now Clinical Cardiology) until August 1965 when Proudfit succeeded him. The following year Van Ordstrand succeeded Ernstene as Chairman of the Division of Medicine, and Ernstene was named Senior Consultant in the Department of Cardiovascular Disease until he retired in 1967.

In 1971 Ernstene sustained a myocardial infarction. [10] He began to have chest pain one night and called Proudfit about 6:30 am, waiting to be sure Proudfit would be awake. Ernstene made his own diagnosis and Proudfit agreed. Refusing to go to the hospital in an ambulance Proudfit drove him and he was admitted to the Clinic's new Coronary Intensive Care unit. He declined to undergo a coronary arteriogram, there being no doubt about the diagnosis, and having no enthusiasm for surgical treatment. A few days later he proclaimed to Proudfit, "This is about it," and died quietly at age 69 on March 12, 1971.[6]

During his thirty-nine years at the Clinic Ernstene received many honors and awards including honorary degrees from John Carroll University and Baldwin Wallace College and the Gold Heart Award of the American Heart Association in 1964. He authored more than a hundred papers on the erythrocytic sedimentation rate and various aspects of cardiovascular disease. Although he never returned to original research after he arrived at the clinic and although he never particularly encouraged research by his staff, he never discouraged it.

He was a pioneer and an esteemed leader in cardiology in Cleveland as well as nationally. Under his leadership four Clinic departments were spawned: Cardiology (the former departments of Clinical Cardiology and Cardiovascular Disease and the Cardiac Laboratory), Pulmonary Disease, Hypertension and Nephrology, and Vascular Medicine. He was beloved by his students and an inspiration to his colleagues.

Notes to The Ernstene Years

1. Rowland[2] states that Ernstene was appointed to the professional staff at the Clinic in November 1929, ten months before Haden arrived. Ernstene's curriculum vitae and other Clinic records indicate that he started in September 1932.
2. The American Board of Internal Medicine was established in 1936. Cardiology was not recognized as a specialty until later. Cardiovascular Disease was established as a subspecialty under the American Board of Internal Medicine in 1941.
3. Later, Proudfit recalled:[6]

> Not long after I returned to the Clinic we had an electrocardiogram that seemed outside the limits of textbook description and my experience. The apparent Q-T interval was very long and the U waves seemed to be fused into the T waves. I checked the chart of this patient in the hospital and found that an extremely low serum potassium had been reported. In those days, potassium was measured by gravimetric analysis that required two days and was done in the Research Building. I went over the laboratory books and found low serum potassium in a number of patients. Electrocardiograms had been done in some of these and most of them showed abnormalities similar to our current case. Oral potassium salts were given to that patient and the ECG returned to normal. Soon the flame photometer became available and rapid determination of potassium was possible. A series of patients having low serum potassium was collected and the ECG's were studied. If the serum level dropped below 3.2 mEq changes in the ECG were demonstrable, although the changes were more dramatic at lower levels. Ernstene was impressed and he and I wrote a paper on hypokalemic abnormalities in the ECG. He wrote the paper, but I did the investigation. He presented a summary of our findings at a meeting of the Association of American Physicians, and it was well received. This was the last scientific paper that Carl wrote. He published other papers but none on original investigation. I extended my interest to hyperkalemia and showed that the serum level of potassium could be predicted with fair precision if the level exceeded 7.0

mEq. This interested Willem Kolff who was treating many renal failure patients with dialysis.

4. Shirey recalls:

    Westcott also had training in cardiac catheterization while at Cincinnati General. One day when I was studying an infant, the catheter traversed a patent foramen ovale and left atrium and entered a pulmonary vein where it became lodged, due to severe spasm of the vessel. The catheter could not be dislodged. Sones was unavailable. Lucile Vanderwyst recalled that Westcott knew something about catheterization and mentioned this to Shirey. Westcott was called and responded immediately. When advised of the dilemma Westcott recommended "Pull the hell out of it!" After a ferocious tug the catheter came free and the patient seemed none the worse. The next day a chest x-ray revealed a local infiltrate in the lung adjacent to the heart where a small extravasation of blood had occurred from the pulmonary vein.[27]

5. After a few encounters I learned to treat Effler's cryptic comments with a humorous rejoinder and he was not offended. In fact, we became friends and in later years we enjoyed each others' company on speaking engagements.
6. Kolff performed the first hemodialysis in 1943 in Kampen, during WW II. After arriving at the Clinic he started working on a disposable artificial kidney, a device for which he later gave the rights to Baxter Travenol.
7. The first open heart operation was done in 1953 by John Heysham Gibbon of Jefferson Medical College with a rotating disc oxygenator.
8. In January 1956 surgeons Bud Kay and Frederick Cross performed Cleveland's first and the world's third open heart operation at St. Vincent Charity Hospital with a rotating disc oxygenator. (Kay EB, Zimmerman HA, Cross FS. Direct-vision intracardiac surgery for pulmonary stenosis. JAMA 1956, (October 6) 162: 563-564.)
9. After Kolff left the Clinic in 1967 for the University of Utah he continued his pioneering work and the Jarvik heart evolved. Under Yukihiko Nose an artificial heart program continued at the Clinic leading to a demonstration in 1976 that a calf could be kept alive for

five months with a total artificial heart—limited only by the animal outgrowing the physiologic capacity of the device, tethered to an extracorporeal drive. Thereafter attention was turned to developing a totally implantable artificial heart, first with implantable assist devices, and later externally powered portable left ventricular assist devices, employed clinically as a bridge to cardiac transplantation.

10. It may be of interest to some that virtually all of these early leaders in cardiovascular disease—Ernstene, Page, Westcott, Whitman, Sones, Effler and Lewis—were smokers. Shirey was only an occasional pipe or cigar smoker and Proudfit never smoked.

References to The Ernstene Years

1. Rourke, MD, Ernstene, AC: A Method for Correcting the Erythrocyte Sedimentation Rate for Variations in the Cell Volume Percentage of Blood. J. Clin. Invest., 1930, 8(4) 545-559.

2. Rowland, A. *Cleveland Clinic Foundation*. Cleveland: William Feather Co; 1938.

3. Bunts, AT and Crile, G Jr: *To Act As a Unit, the Story of the Cleveland Clinic*. Cleveland: The Cleveland Clinic; 1971.

4. Proudfit WL: Notes on A. Carlton Ernstene M.D. Unpublished, 1971.

5. Hartwell, SW Editor. *". . . to act as a unit" the Story of the Cleveland Clinic*. 2nd edition. Philadelphia: WB Saunders; 1985.

6. Proudfit WL: Unpublished conversations with the author. April, 2005.

7. Ernstene AC and Levine SA: Observations on arterial blood pressure during attacks of angina. Am Heart J. 1933;8:323.

8. Dustan HP, Page IH, Poutasse EF: Renal hypertension. N Engl J Med. 1959; Sep 24;261:647-53.

9. Page IH, Bumpus FM: Angiotensin. Physiol Rev. 1961; Apr;41:331-90.

10. Page IH, Dustan HP: A new, potent antihypertensive drug: preliminary study of [2-(octahydro-1-azocinyl)-ethyl]-guanidine sulfate (guanethidine). J Am Med Assoc. 1959; Jul 11;170(11):1265-71.

11. Brown HB, Page IH: Lowering blood lipid levels by changing food patterns. J Am Med Assoc. 1958; Dec 13;168(15):1989-95.

12. Abbott ME: A statistical study and historical retrospect of 200 recorded cases, with autopsy, of stenosis or obliteration of the descending arch in subjects above the age of two years. Am Heart J. 1928; 3:92.

13. Gross ER and Hubbard JP: Surgical ligation of patent ductus arteriosus: report of first successful case. JAMA. 1939;112:729.

14. Abbott, Maude E.: Atlas of Congenital Heart Disease. New York: American Heart Association; 1936.

15. Gross RE: Surgical therapy for the patent ductus arteriosus. New York J Med. 1943;43:1856.

16. Blalock A and Park EA: Surgical treatment of coarctation (atresia) of aorta. Ann Surg. 1944;128:803.

17. Blalock A and Taussig HB: Surgical treatment of malformations of the heart in which there is pulmonary stenosis or pulmonary atresia. JAMA. 1945;128:189.

18. Forssman W: Die Sondierung des Rechten Herzens. Klin Wochenschr. 1929;8:2085-2087.

19. Cournand A and Ranges HA: Catheterization of the right auricle in man. Proc Soc Exper Biol & Med. 1941;46:462-466.

20. Sones, FM Jr, Effler, DB: Diagnosis and treatment of aortic rings. Cleve Clin Q. 1951;18:310-320.

21. Favaloro RG: *The challenging dream of heart surgery. From Pampus to Cleveland.* Cleveland: The Cleveland Clinic Foundation; 1992.

22. Academy of Achievement. Interview with Willem J. Kolff, M.D. November 15, 1991. http://www.achievement.org/autodoc/page/kol0int-1. Revised Feb 05, 2005, copyright 2006, accessed July 26, 2006.

23. Kolff WJ, Effler DB, Groves LK, et al: Disposable membrane oxygenator (heart-lung machine) and its use in experimental surgery. Cleve Clin Q. 1956;Apr; 23(2):69-97.

24. Kolff WJ, Effler DB, Groves LK, et al: Elective cardiac arrest by the Melrose technic: potassium asystole for experimental cardiac surgery. Cleve Clin Q. 1956;Apr; 23(2):98-104.

25. Effler DB, Groves LK, Sones FM Jr, Kolff, WJ: Elective cardiac arrest in open heart surgery: Report of three cases. Cleve Clin Q. 1956;Apr; 23(2):105-114.

26. Clough JD Editor *". . . to act as a unit"* The Story of the Cleveland Clinic, 3rd edition, Cleveland: The Cleveland Clinic; 1996.

27. Shirey EK: Unpublished conversation with the author, October 2006.

THE PROUDFIT-SONES YEARS

Sones: 1960-1975
Proudfit: 1965-1974

In 1955 Sones' clinic in the Section of Pediatric Cardiology was at Desk 81, but he had relocated his office to the third floor of the old Clinic building to be near the Cardiac Catheterization Laboratory. In the outpatient department, Sones routinely fluoroscoped his young patients as a part of their initial evaluation, and he taught cardiac fluoroscopy to others. In the catheterization laboratory only right heart catheterizations were performed in the early years, and the left ventricle was entered across a patent foramen ovale or interatrial septal defect. In 1955 he began to study infants and children with newly developed cineangiographic equipment. He learned about image amplifiers from Dr. Russell H. Morgan at Johns Hopkins University. The first image intensifiers had a five-inch output screen that was viewed with a reflecting mirror periscope. The image could be reflected in two directions that allowed the operator and an assistant to watch the process. Of necessity Sones became expert in radiographic technology, and, working with the Eastman Kodak Co., he also learned about photographic lens systems, motion picture film and film processing. He also learned about film editing, and contrast media.

Sones studied infants and adults from cutdowns over the saphenous or superficial femoral vein, and the superficial femoral artery. [1] Dr. Henry Zimmerman at St. Vincent Charity Hospital had introduced retrograde left heart catheterizations in 1950.[1] [2] Contrast injections were photographed with a 16mm motion picture camera using the 5-inch image amplifier that had just been installed. Patients were sedated, but general anesthesia was never used. Among the fellows who worked with Sones in the early years were Eric Kemp, Frank LeCamera, Grace Hofsteter, and later Roy Lewis.

Fellows were taught to do the cutdowns and wound closures. The fellows' job was also to control the X-ray exposure to maintain a steady brightness of the amplifier's image as the image intensifier was moved about the chest during the cine-exposures, in order to avoid over—or underexposure of the motion picture film. (The kilovolt potential to the X-ray tube was fixed; the milliampere current was variable and controlled by the fellow, monitoring a light meter from the image intensifier at the control counsel). Fellows also were needed to help restrain rebellious infants and children. Sones would not allow general anesthesia or deep sedation. Fellows learned cardiac catheterization by watching Sones, observing catheter technique via a mirror periscope that reflected the view from the image intensifier, and in sitting by his side as he dictated his interpretation of the cines. In due course they were allowed hands-on catheter time.

The cardiac catheterization laboratory was moved to a larger space in the basement of the Clinic building, "B-10," in 1958. Earl K. Shirey, who joined Sones in 1956 as a special fellow, was appointed to the Staff in the Department of Cardiorespiratory Disease (Section of Pediatric Cardiology and the Cardiac Laboratory) in January 1957. Although Sones' laboratory was not yet a separate department, it functioned more or less independently. Shirey became an expert in cardiac catheterization and in congenital heart disease.

Earl Shirey looked like a TV physician, although he did not drape a stethoscope across his shoulders. He was handsome and immaculate in appearance whether in his office or the laboratory. He is the soul of modesty. Earl never seemed hurried but handled duties rapidly. He treated patients in a way that they hoped their physician would.

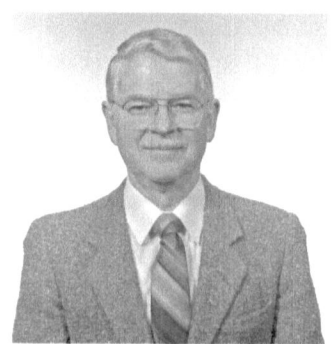

Earl K. Shirey

Despite his training in pharmacy, he disdained unnecessary use of drugs. Earl was courteous to patients, Clinic personnel, nurses, technicians, residents in training and colleagues. He had a good background in internal medicine and treated the whole patient. Shirey was intelligent but never talked down to patients.

Shirey proved to be a blessing for Mason Sones who soon learned that he was responsible for much of the smooth running of the Department.

Few others could have lived with Sones for many years without friction. He was completely loyal to Sones and became his right hand man. He soon became recognized as one of the Clinic's outstanding teachers.

With the advent of open-heart surgery in the mid 1950's increasing numbers of patients with complex congenital heart disease were referred for surgery. Initially the surgical mortality in patients with congenital heart disease, many of whom were high-risk, was 30%. Effler attributed this to pulmonary vascular disease that was recognizable on the chest x-ray. Sones disagreed and believed the high mortality was due to poor surgical technique. One day, to debate the issue, a special meeting of surgical and cardiology fellows was arranged. Sones presented chest x-rays of patients with and without severe pulmonary hypertension and Effler was to identify those with pulmonary vascular disease. It became clear that Effler could not reliably identify pulmonary vascular disease from the chest x-rays. "Closed" mitral commissurotomy was the treatment for rheumatic mitral stenosis[2,3] until after 1956 when open-heart technics were introduced. Aortic valvotomies for rheumatic aortic stenosis were tried but were never particularly successful.

It was about this time that Sones, Effler and Kolff became involved in the conflicts for which Proudfit had been called to mediate. Sones attended the operating rooms and observed the surgical procedures done on many of his patients, criticizing the surgeons' every move. He made rounds on his patients personally each day, including Effler's and Groves' postoperative patients. He was a difficult taskmaster, finding fault with the surgeons, the floor nurses, and nearly everyone else. Some nurses would hide in a bathroom when Sones appeared on the floor. It was not long before the Board of Governors intervened and instructed Sones to delegate the hospital coverage of his patients to someone else, and Shirey was the obvious candidate. With Shirey managing the hospital service it ran much more smoothly.

As patients with rheumatic heart disease were referred for mitral commissurotomies, Sones and Shirey catheterized more adults. Sones became intrigued with visualization of coronary arteries during aortograms, and experimented with selective opacification of right or left sinuses of Valsalva to achieve better opacification. He became disenchanted with the five-inch image amplifier. Although too large even for the smallest infants, it was thought to be too small for the increasing numbers of adults being studied. The North American Philips Corporation developed an 11-inch image amplifier that Sones thought would be more useful, especially for adults. This instrument was very large—six feet long, and heavy—over 600 pounds, and could not be mounted vertically with the input phosphor at the bottom, because its metal case was soldered together, and flecks of solder from the casing would fall upon the input phosphor degrading the image. It therefore had to be installed upside-down, beneath the table—all six feet of it—with the x-ray tube above the patient. In excavating a pit beneath the basement floor that would accommodate the 11-inch amplifier, water was encountered, from a creek that ran beneath the Clinic building. This was a complication that required major reconstruction—at a reported cost of $150,000—before the installation could be completed. [3]

The First Coronary Arteriogram

In 1958 Royston Lewis was a fellow rotating through the catheterization laboratory as a part of a special fellowship funded by the U.S. Public Health Service. On October 30, 1958 Sones was studying a twenty-six year old man from West Virginia with rheumatic mitral and aortic valve disease, with Lewis assisting, and Lucile Vanderwyst as the circulating nurse. After completing a left ventriculogram he prepared to perform an aortogram. He positioned the closed-tip catheter in the ascending aorta just above the aortic valve and loaded the Gidlund pressure injector with 50

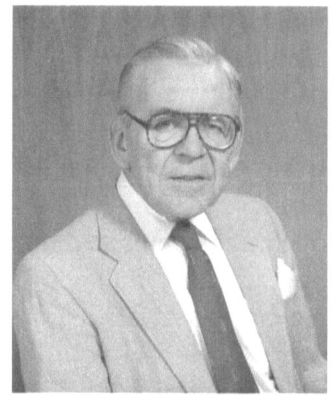

Royston C. Lewis

ml. of contrast material. With Lewis at the patient's side, his hand on the catheter, Sones climbed down into the pit next to the 11-inch amplifier where he could control the motion picture camera and visually monitor the aortogram. Activating the camera, he gave the order for Lewis to fire the injector. To his horror, as he watched, most of the contrast material injected, approximately 30 ml, was delivered directly into the right coronary artery heavily opacifying it. [4] He frantically ordered Lewis to "Pull it out!" but by then it was too late.

Conventional wisdom at that time, promulgated by Claude Beck, a cardiac surgeon at Western Reserve University Medical School, was that any medium other than blood that was injected directly into one coronary artery would create not only ischemia, but an electrically unstable interface with tissue perfused by the opposite coronary artery, and ventricular fibrillation would ensue. Sones leaped up from the pit and shoving Lewis aside grabbed a scalpel from the instrument table to open the chest and perform open cardiac massage. However he noted that the patient was still conscious. He glanced at the ECG monitor that showed marked sinus bradycardia which led to asystole for five seconds, not the ventricular fibrillation he had expected. Impulsively he ordered the patient, whose consciousness was waning, to "cough!" A slow sinus rhythm returned and then in a few seconds, a normal sinus rhythm.

Perplexed by the sight of Sones, scalpel in hand, poised to attack him, the patient recovered fully within a minute. Sones had previously explored contrast visualization of coronary arteries in dogs with aortic root injections of contrast material. With this event he immediately recognized the potential for selective opacification of coronary arteries in humans and noted this in his catheterization report that was dictated that day:

> This is the first instance in which we have seen extremely heavy opacification of a single coronary vessel with contrast media. This potential complication had been feared to result in a ventricular arrhythmia due to the development of asymmetrical hypoxia in the coronary circulation. Its failure to occur inder this extreme asymmetrical injection of 90% Hypaque where at least 30 cc. of the media passed directly into the artery with absolutely no opacification of the left coronary artery is a source of considerable satisfaction regarding the further diagnostic evolution of this technique.

When Sones and Shirey reported their experience with coronary arteriography at the meeting of the American Heart Association in 1959 their series included more than fifty patients.[4] In this report Sones curiously described "selective opacification" as injections of 20-30 ml into the right or left sinuses of Valsalva, with no complications. They had observed normal coronary arteries in patients with chest pain syndromes, partial or total occlusions of coronary arteries, and intercoronary collaterals. They concluded, modestly, that

> The ultimate usefulness of the method remains to be defined, but it should provide a more objective diagnostic standard than has previously been available for the evaluation of therapeutic measures which have been or may be applied in the treatment of arteriosclerotic heart disease.[4]

After the event of October 1958 Sones discussed the potential of selective coronary arteriography with Ernstene who listened intently, then replied, "Go ahead as long as you don't hurt anyone." There were no institutional review boards in the 1950's. He began deliberately to opacify coronary arteries of patients referred to him for study of their rheumatic heart disease. He replaced the 11-inch image amplifier with a 5-inch instrument and prevailed upon David Prigmore of the U.S. Catheter and Instrument Co. to develop a catheter with a special tapered flexible tip that would facilitate catheterization of the coronary arteries. Thus began a relationship with USCI that led to its enormously profitable virtual monopoly on coronary artery catheters (both before and after its merger with Bard in 1966, and its later acquisition of rights from the Schneider Company to manufacture and sell the Grüntzig's balloon angioplasty catheter in the U.S.A.) Sones relationship with Philips was also legendary. Working with Fred Lignon and William Angus, M.D. of Philips, the technology of X-ray image amplification and cine angiography evolved rapidly, and Philips became the pacesetter among X-ray equipment manufacturers. [5]

A Second Cardiology Department

Although William L Proudfit preceded Sones at the Clinic by four years when he joined the Department of Cardiorespiratory Disease under Ernstene in 1946, Sones was appointed Chairman of the new Department of Pediatric Cardiology and the Cardiac Laboratory in 1960, five years before Proudfit succeeded Ernstene as Chairman of Clinical Cardiology in 1965. However they had become close friends and had great respect for each other personally and professionally.

By 1958 Proudfit became interested in electrocardiographic monitoring. Working with an engineer friend, Joe Dobosy, he developed one of the earliest tape recording electrocardiographs. They were able to record eight hours continuously, and view the exact moment of conversion of various arrhythmias to sinus rhythm. Dobosy

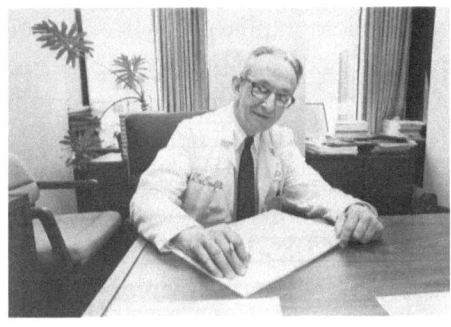

also devised a large screen display of multiple electrocardiograms for continuous monitoring in the hospital setting. The small "bullet" bedside monitors used at that time were helpful only if a nurse was stationed at the bedside. Proudfit promoted the large screen monitors which could be viewed from a distance—i.e. in the nursing station. He was ahead of his time however, as coronary intensive care units were not to come into practice nationally until 1963, and at the Clinic, 1970.

As Sones and Shirey gained experience with coronary arteriography their confidence and enthusiasm grew. When they reported their work at a meeting of the American Heart Association in November 1959, and the report appeared in abstract form in *Circulation,*[4] this author was a resident in internal medicine in Chicago. Local cardiologists looked upon Sones as a maverick. When I interviewed for a fellowship at the Clinic in the spring of 1960, although a patient was waiting for him in the cath lab, Sones grabbed an armful of films and spent about an hour with me in a fourth floor conference room enthusiastically showing me cineangiograms on a 16 mm projector, illustrating what he had learned from coronary arteriography. Suddenly he remembered that a patient was waiting and he hurried back to the lab. By the time I arrived in Cleveland in July 1960 Sones and Shirey had done more than 600 coronary arteriograms.

External Cardiac Compression and Defibrillation

In June 1960 Sones invited Michael Criley of Johns Hopkins University to visit his Laboratory. He was interested in developing a photographic format for catheterization reports, and Criley was an experienced amateur photographer. He showed Sones and Adam Benowski, his cine-processing technician, how to make photographic prints from selected frames of the 35 mm cineangiograms, process them, and incorporate them into the report. Sones added a descriptive caption for each, creating a report that was both educational and informative for referring physicians. One day when Criley was observing a coronary arteriogram, the patient developed ventricular fibrillation after an intracoronary injection of contrast. As Sones prepared to open the patient's chest to massage the heart, Criley interceded, and showed Sones a technique that had been used at Johns Hopkins by a senior researcher, William Kouwenhoven, closed chest cardiac massage.[5] Each chest compression indeed produced a measurable pressure pulse on the pressure monitor and the patient remained conscious. [6] It provided support for sufficient time for the patient to be transferred to the operating room where the chest could be opened under more controlled circumstances, and the heart internally defibrillated. That was the last time that internal defibrillation was necessary. Until then, three patients had required open cardiac massage and internal defibrillation, two of whom died and one survived after a stormy postoperative course. Weeks later a Zoll AC external cardiac defibrillator was delivered and the combination of closed chest massage and external defibrillation were almost uniformly successful for treating contrast induced ventricular fibrillation. It was not long before the AC defibrillator was replaced with a DC defibrillator. This defibrillator could also be programmed to discharge at any designated point in the heart cycle, which led to elective "cardioversion" of atrial arrhythmias including atrial fibrillation, accomplished under brief intravenous anesthesia—initially delivered by anesthesiologists, later by the attending cardiologist. (I remember when Carl Wiggers, a renowned cardiovascular physiologist working in the Research Division of the Clinic, came to the laboratory in the summer of 1960 to observe an elective defibrillation.)

Although Sones always wrote with precision, writing for publication was a task he abhorred, fearing that he would be misinterpreted. His first detailed experience with coronary arteriography was not reported until 1962 when it was invited by the editors of *Modern Concepts of Cardiovascular Disease*, a publication of the American Heart Association.[8] By this time he and Shirey had done more than 1020 cases.

In 1960 patients in the Cath Lab were evenly divided between those with congenital heart disease, rheumatic heart disease, and known or suspected coronary heart disease. In the mid 1960s, with the development of a subspecialty board in pediatrics for pediatric cardiologists, the Ohio Services for Crippled Children, which had been the source of many referrals of infants and children with congenital heart disease, began to restrict its referrals to cardiologists that were board certified. Sones, whose training preceded any cardiology boards, had no board certification and he was dropped from the referral list. Shirey was certified in Cardiovascular Disease however, and continued to receive referrals of patients with congenital heart disease. But as valve surgery and coronary arteriography developed, congenital heart disease patients became overshadowed. Later, in 1965, the last key source for referrals for patients with congenital heart disease disappeared when the obstetrical service and neonatal unit on the sixth floor of the hospital were closed to make way for the expansion of cardiac surgery.

Coronary arteriography led to many new observations by Sones and his colleagues: spasm of coronary arteries, spontaneous coronary dissection, "myocardial bridges" (systolic narrowing of an epicardial segment of a coronary artery, usually the anterior descending), the "septal squeeze" of IHSS (systolic narrowing or obliteration of septal perforating branches of the anterior descending coronary artery in idiopathic subaortic stenosis), the "septal dance" of left bundle branch block, the diastolic "shudder" of constrictive pericarditis (the sudden cessation of expansile motion of the coronary arteries in mid diastole due to restricted filling of the left ventricle), mitral valve prolapse, and hundreds of anatomical variations and congenital coronary anomalies. Increasingly Sones and Shirey were invited to other institutions, regional and national meetings, and soon internationally, to talk about coronary arteriography and show their movies, which by now they were adept at making. When they encountered an interesting abnormality or congenital variation, they would have 16 mm copies made of the 35 mm film, and file the copies and catalog them in an extensive film library in a back room of the laboratory at B-10. They created a cine-indexing system and built a film library that contained examples of every conceivable manifestation of coronary artery anatomy and pathology including congenital variations, as well as valvular and other cardiac abnormalities. This would become the world's largest and most comprehensive angiographic library of cardiac pathology. [7]

Whenever Sones attended a national meeting he would return with a cadre of cardiologists whom he invited to visit and observe. Although he hated to write, and rarely read medical literature, he was a great communicator and loved to talk, especially about his work, and would spend hours with his visitors, usually late into the evening. He listened intently to what visitors had to say which is how he learned about medical advances. He was always open to new ideas, but quick to perceive a sham. As he grew older he became more emotional and tears came easily, at the slightest provocation, even during his talks and panel discussions. Those who knew him understood this peculiarity and learned to be patient, and that he would soon compose himself.

Typically the fellows would see Sones' and Shirey's patients first in the outpatient department. After the staff physician saw the patient, he or she was admitted to the hospital overnight. Sones would have from two to five cases scheduled the next day in the laboratory; his cases were always scheduled to be first in the morning although he rarely arrived on time having been out late with a visitor the evening before. The fellow would do the cutdown, and right heart catheterization if indicated. Sones would be called when the patient was ready. He was also frequently delayed when he became involved talking with a visitor in his office. He would appear in the laboratory smoking a cigarette and wearing a V-neck T-shirt under the lead X-ray apron. A fellow operated the X-ray controls to maintain a steady light meter reading from the image intensifier for optimal angiographic image quality, and the nurse operated the pressure/ECG recorder, the pressure injector, and changed film canisters when needed. He rarely scrubbed, but donned sterile gloves. Often Sones would smoke during the procedure, and, using a sterile forceps, park the lighted cigarette on the edge of the instrument table. When finished Sones would report the findings briefly to the patient and leave.

The fellow would close the incision and write the post-cath orders. The cineangiograms were developed within an hour or two, and Sones would view them and dictate a detailed report personally. He set the example that everyone dictate their catheterization reports on the day of the procedure. (Later his fellow would dictate the first part of the report—the history, physical, laboratory, ECG and X-ray findings,—leaving the angiographic details for Sones to dictate). He would see his patients the next day—between cases, for a final report and recommendations—and they often waited long periods of time. Shirey and the fellows would see his hospital patients and report to him. He rarely had lunch—or perhaps only snack in his office. In the evenings he would spend time with visitors, or make movies for upcoming presentations.

Proudfit recalls another characteristic vignette:

> One day as I walked into his office, Sones' secretary was laughing about an incident that had occurred shortly before. [8] Donald Ross (a little later Sir Donald), a surgeon at the National Heart Hospital in London, had called Mason. The secretary said, "I am sorry, Dr. Ross, but Dr. Sones has just left his office to do a coronary arteriogram." Mr. Ross answered, "Please ask him to call me when he is free." The secretary retorted, "If you can hold on for a couple of minutes, he will be with you." Ross was astonished to hear Mason's voice in two or three minutes after Sones had completed his procedure.[9]

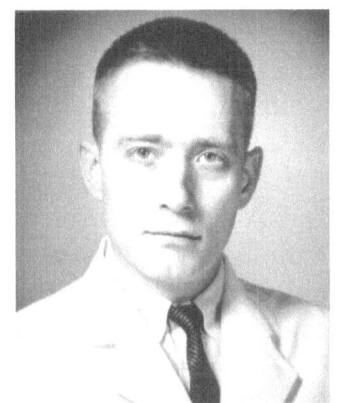

William C. Sheldon

William Sheldon was born in Elkhorn, Wisconsin and attended Northwestern University Medical School. After completing an internship and internal medicine residency in Chicago, and a two-year rotating U.S. Public Health Service Fellowship at the Clinic in 1962, he joined the Department of Cardiovascular Disease and the Cardiac Laboratory as a Clinical Associate and was appointed Assistant Staff the following year. [9] When Sones discussed joining the Staff he told him that this group practice was unique, and that "you'll never make more than $25,000." All were expected to "put in more than (you) take out." Sheldon had always planned to return to Chicago which was closer to home, but after discussing the prospect with his wife, Margaret, they decided to stay in Cleveland and give it a try for five years or so. Five years later they never revisited that decision.

In about 1963 Sones' mother experienced atypical chest pain, and he performed a coronary arteriogram, finding no significant disease. Some criticized him for doing his. Sometime later he experienced chest discomfort himself. A friend of Sones, Don Nouse of Toledo, recalled:

> One early morning about 6:15 am, I received a call as I was coming to Toledo Hospital. Mason was on the other end of the line and he said "I'm having some chest pain what would you

do about it if it were you?" and I said "I'd do the same thing you would tell me to do and that's get your butt down to the cardiac laboratory and have the best person you know inject your coronaries and see what they show." Not more than a half hour later he called me back and said "You little SOB they're normal, now what would you do?" and I said, "Quit smoking!" and hung up. About half an hour later Mason called me back and he said "You smart SOB you know I'm never going to give that up and I'm going to live with my chest pain."[10]

He had Shirey perform the coronary arteriogram. During the course of the study he developed severe spasm of the right coronary artery, and Shirey, never betraying his concern, said nothing. Sones had no symptoms and the spasm subsided promptly after the customary administration of a nitroglycerin tablet. He subsequently used that angiogram in many of his talks.

One August afternoon in 1963 while reviewing cines in Sones' office, a triple page call was received from 2-West. The patient was a 66-year-old woman, the mother of Lucile Vanderwyst, the head nurse in the catheterization laboratory, who had been admitted to the hospital the previous day with acute coronary insufficiency. Sones, Marshall Franklin, and William Sheldon, both Clinical Associates in the Department, ran at breakneck speed from B-10 and up four flights of stairs to find her on the floor, cyanotic and pulseless, in full cardiac arrest, and the house staff was applying closed chest massage. At that time cardiac defibrillators had not yet become standard components of "crash carts" and one had to be obtained from another part of the hospital while Sones and colleagues continued external cardiac massage. Once obtained, the A-C defibrillator was set up, and with its first discharge promptly blew a fuse and the entire wing of the floor was suddenly without power. The patient was still in ventricular fibrillation. With an agonizing delay another defibrillator was located and connected to an outlet in an adjoining wing with a long extension cord, a second shock was applied. A transient idioventricular rhythm deteriorated to asystole, but after prolonged closed chest massage and repeated shocks a slow idioventricular rhythm was obtained, then atrial fibrillation. This was before coronary intensive care units were in vogue, (the first coronary intensive care unit at the Clinic was not until 1970, a four-bed unit on 4-East directed by Royston Lewis.) and Franklin and

Sheldon "specialed" the patient for the next 24 hours. Mrs. Vanderwyst remained in a coma for two days, but miraculously she began to respond, ultimately becoming lucid and regaining all her faculties. Coronary arteriography three weeks later revealed total occlusion of the anterior descending artery and an anterolateral ventricular aneurysm. She lived for eleven years after that, limited only by her arthritis and advancing age, before she succumbed to a gastrointestinal hemorrhage at age 77.

Always an innovator, in October 1959 Sones attempted to dissolve a fresh thrombus in a 43 year old man with an acute inferior myocardial infarction by infusing streptokinase directly into the stenosed right coronary artery. In July 1964 he attempted to dilate a stenosed right coronary artery of a 45 year old man with a catheter guidewire (stylus), and a catheter. With Lowell Edwards he developed a "rotorooter" catheter to drill through occluded coronary artery segments. Working with North American Philips Corp. in the early 1970s he explored stereoscopic coronary arteriography using twin X-ray tubes, each pulsed and synchronized to expose alternate frames of 35mm cine film, and viewed with a special "clicker" device, that was electrically coupled with the Taj Arno projector, and designed to transmit alternate images from the Taj Arno projector to either eye. The brain fused the images if viewed rapidly enough and three dimensions were perceived. [10] With Philips he also explored electron beam angiography, an alternative to image amplifiers. He also designed a hand-held power injector to facilitate contrast injections into the coronary arteries. [11] He disliked gadgets, however, unless they proved to have a useful purpose.

In the early 1970's there was a sudden increase in the incidence of ventricular fibrillation with intracoronary injections of contrast material. Sones examined the contrast material, and comparing the new bottles with the old, observed that a small but definite change in the concentration of sodium had been made—which had never been announced by the manufacturer. Sones called the corporate headquarters and learned that indeed this change had occurred in the manufacturing process. He returned to using an older supply of the contrast agent and immediately the incidence of ventricular fibrillation fell to the usual modest level. At that point Sones again called the manufacturer with a scathing criticism, and he called or wrote to every angiographer that he knew informing them of his experience and warning them not to use the newly supplied contrast agent.

The manufacturer immediately recalled the offending agent and returned to the original manufacturing process. Sones never wrote publicly of this experience, nor did the manufacturer.

In the early 1960s, after Sones had been banned from hospital rounds, Shirey and Sheldon shared hospital rounds. Patients were admitted to the hospital on what came to be known as the Sones-Shirey-Sheldon (S-S-S) Service. On alternate days each worked in the catheterization laboratory. Each morning Shirey and Sheldon would meet with the fellows to review the status of hospital patients. As new staff were added to the Department and the number of hospital patients increased, it became more difficult to see them all on rounds in the morning, and finish in time to begin seeing patients that were scheduled in the outpatient clinic in the afternoon. In later years the S-S-S system was abandoned and each catheterizing cardiologist rounded on his own patients daily, and Sones' hospital patients were divided among the other Department staff members.

During these years Sones had insisted that his Department fully support Cardiac Surgery. In the early days of catheterization the surgeons had always been responsive whenever problems occurred in the cath lab. Effler and colleagues were eager for referrals of infants and children with congenital heart disease evaluated by Sones and Shirey. The departments became mutually dependent upon one another. As the practice grew all patients who were potential candidates for surgery, children and adults, were referred to a staff member in either of the two cardiology departments for evaluation. After catheterization, those who were surgical candidates were then referred to one of the cardiac surgeons, selected either by the outside referring physician or the Clinic cardiologist. Postoperative care became a shared responsibility between the Clinic surgeons and cardiologists (other than Sones), the surgeons managing the immediate care in the intensive care unit including wound issues and fluids, the cardiologists managing the medical care, arrhythmias, homegoing medications and discharge instructions. After the patient was discharged routine six-week followup visits were done by the cardiologist who had seen the patient preoperatively (or sometimes the outside referring physician), and the cardiologist was usually responsible for the annual long-term followup visits. This allowed the surgeons to devote nearly full attention to operating, and the cardiologist became the attending physician, communicating with the patients and their families and outside referring physicians.

The arrangement worked well, and contributed to quality care and optimal surgical results. Each patient always had a specific cardiologist as his primary Clinic physician, one upon whom he or she, or his or her outside personal physician, could call if there were problems. It was the private practice model that other Clinic Departments had followed and had contributed to the growth of the Clinic. It was the "town" model and antithesis of the "town and gown" conflict that began to emerge in medical schools a decade earlier.

Valve Replacement and Direct Coronary Surgery

The first valve replacements at the Clinic were performed in 1962, using Starr-Edwards prostheses, first in the mitral position, later in the aortic position. Also, in January 1962, Effler began performing direct coronary surgery with endarterectomy and patch graft reconstruction. It was quickly learned that operative risk was high for direct operations on the left coronary artery or its branches, but results for the right coronary artery were encouraging. [12]

The Vineberg Procedure

In January and March 1962 Sones had the opportunity to study two patients who had been operated upon five years earlier, one by Vineberg, the other by Bigelow, using Vineberg's internal mammary implantation for myocardial revascularization. Vineberg's work had not been generally accepted as validation of the procedure had been accomplished only by India ink injections of post-mortem implants, and patients were selected on purely clinical, rather than anatomical criteria. Sones was surprised to observe that contrast material injected into an implanted internal mammary artery showed small channels that produced a myocardial "blush" with subsequent opacification of the coronary venous system. This was the first *in vivo* confirmation of myocardial perfusion from internal mammary implants. Sones showed the angiograms to Effler who was willing to perform such a procedure if Sones would provide the patient. The first internal mammary implant procedure at the Clinic was done by Effler in April 1962.[11] Left internal mammary inplants were used for left coronary disease, and right coronary endarterectomies were sometimes combined with internal mammary implants when there was associated disease in the right coronary system.

Postoperative angiograms within the first few months showed patency of most of the implants, but no definite myocardial perfusion. Thereafter postoperative study of these patients was deferred for a year or more, when they showed patency with evidence of myocardial perfusion in about 70 percent of cases. There were limitations however, in that the standard Vineberg procedure was useful only for patients with anterior descending disease, and the symptomatic improvement was slow, with the gradual development of new intramyocardial channels. Later the technique was modified by implanting the internal mammary artery into both the anterior and posterolateral aspects of the left ventricle—the anteroposterior or "A-P" implant, the use of the internal mammary pedicle with its contiguous soft tissue as a graft instead of the bare artery, the use of the right internal mammary artery for the posterior aspect of the left ventricle, and finally the use of bilateral internal mammary implants.[12]

Thus began the era of myocardial revascularization surgery, and a period of unprecedented growth of the Cleveland Clinic. [13]

The Favaloro Era

In February 1962, Rene Favaloro, a 38-year old aspiring cardiac surgeon from Argentina arrived in Cleveland hoping to become a fellow in Cardiac Surgery under Effler. His mentor, Professor Jose' Maria Mainetti, had previously written to Dr. George Crile Jr. on two occasions but had received no response. [14] Favaloro was unexpected. Effler sent him to the Director of Education Division, Dr. Charles Leedham, who summarily rejected him having had an unfortunate experience with another surgical resident from Argentina. Dismayed, Favaloro called Crile who in turn

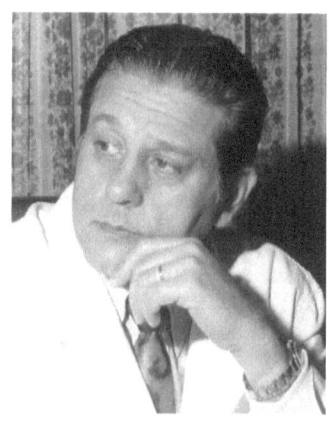

Rene G. Favaloro

prevailed upon Effler to allow him to observe cardiac surgery. Soon Favaloro was a fully credentialed Fellow in the Department and began working with Effler and Groves. He became interested in coronary artery surgery. Favaloro wandered into Mason Sones office one night. He asked Mason for permission to review arteriographic films in the evenings, at a time when few would be inconvenienced. Sones asked about his background and Favaloro related that he was from Argentina, had practiced general surgery there with his brother, also a surgeon, was a vigorous protestor of the dictator Juan Peron and had been advised to "internally exile himself" if he wished to remain free—or perhaps even alive—and that he was an observer in Effler's Department. Sones was impressed and showed him how to use the equipment in the film library. Every evening, after surgery, Favaloro assiduously reviewed films, often working into the very late hours, and learned coronary artery anatomy and its variations in health and disease, with Sones mentoring him like a private student. He was a tireless worker. He and Sones formed a deep and lasting friendship.

Effler quickly recognized Favaloro's surgical skills. When he completed his fellowship in 1965 Effler offered him a position on the staff. However, Favaloro chose to return to Argentina in August 1965 to test the waters for building a career there. But he found the political climate disappointing and returned to Cleveland in December 1966 where he began a career that earned him international recognition.

In November 1963 the American Heart Association held its annual Scientific Session in Cleveland. On the weekend the meeting was to begin Cleveland experienced one of its famous early winter storms with a heavy lake-effect snowfall. The airport was closed for a short time, and hotels remained full with attendees of a previous meeting that week, unable to get flights home. As AHA attendees gradually arrived the meeting proceeded on schedule.

One of the sessions was on coronary arteriography and Sones reported on his experience to date. The moderator, Dr. George Burch of Tulane University School of Medicine, rebutted Sones' presentation, calling coronary arteriography "experimental" and not ready for clinical application. That Sones and the Cleveland Clinic contingent were gravely affronted by Burch's performance was no secret. That was the last time the AHA met in Cleveland. [15]

A second catheterization laboratory had been added in B-10 in 1963. In about 1965 one of a continuing series of postgraduate courses in cardiology was held in the new Bunts Auditorium of the Clinic. With the help of the Philips Corporation a closed circuit television demonstration of catheterization procedures was included—one of the first live demonstrations ever conducted. Fortunately there were no complications.

A third and fourth catheterization laboratories were added in about 1966 along with additional offices to accommodate the growing staff: David Fergusson (1966), Mehdi Razavi (1967), Robert Quint (1968) and Ted Huston and Joel Webster (1969).

David Fergusson was a charismatic young cardiologist from Durbin, South Africa whom Walter Sommerville, a well-known London cardiologist, had met during a visit. At the time the problems of apartheid were unsettling for South Afrikaners and Fergusson was considering a move. Fergusson was well trained and experienced in cardiac catheterization and congenital heart disease. Upon Sommerville's recommendation Sones hired Fergusson without ever having met him.

Mehdi Razavi, a Persian graduate of the University of Isfahan, came to the United States on a special fellowship funded by the Shah of Iran for graduate medical training. After learning English in Washington D.C. he did a residency in Internal Medicine at Akron City Hospital, then Cardiology at the Cleveland Clinic. Although he had been expected to return to Iran to practice medicine, he instead joined the Clinic Staff. He rapidly became "Americanized" and became an excellent, empathetic physician. Traces of his Farsi accent persisted throughout his career.

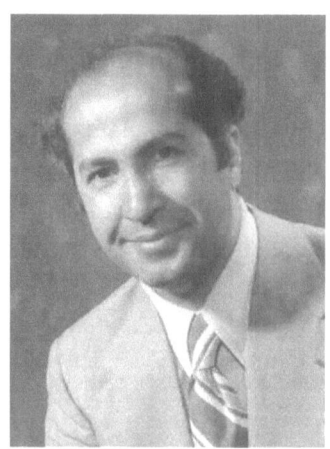
Mehdi Razavi

Robert Quint was a graduate of Ohio State University College of Medicine and residencies in internal medicine and cardiology at the Clinic. Quint and Sones had much in common: both were "night people"—working late into the night and arriving at work late the next morning—as late as 10-11 am. Fellows came to look upon Quint as a great friend and teacher as he was usually available to help them with complicated patient problems in the late evening or early morning hours.

Ted Huston was also a graduate of Ohio State University College of Medicine, with training in internal medicine at Riverside Hospital in Columbus, and cardiology at the Clinic. Huston was a tall easygoing fellow, but very capable. He was the antithesis of Sones and Quint.

Joel Webster had been in practice in Dayton Ohio for several years, and was a regular referrer to the Clinic. He was experienced in cardiac catheterization, and was known and respected by Clinic cardiologists. Somewhat disenchanted with the tribulations of private practice he inquired of Sones about a position and was hired immediately.

In 1968 David Fergusson analyzed postoperative angiograms of internal mammary implant patients and observed that demonstrable myocardial perfusion was most likely occur from an implant if the native coronary artery supplying the region was severely diseased with proximal narrowing exceeding 90 percent, and especially when there were preexisting intercoronary collaterals perfusing the ischemic area.[13,14] (It was also Fergusson who first fashioned a short, acutely angled tip on an extruded Cordis catheter that facilitated selective catheterization of internal mammary arteries. Fergusson was the first in Sones' department to write and publish a report based on angiographic followup. Sones' aborhence of writing had served as a disincentive for his colleagues to independently publish. [16] In conducting his followup studies of surgical patients Fergusson lamented the lack of a registry or database of surgical patients that would have made his work easier).

Sones became a sought after speaker, and traveled the world with cardiology's leaders: Richard Bing, Walter Sommerville, Aubrey Leatham, Harold Dodge, Eliot Corday, Norman Shumway, Richard Gorlin, Jeremy Swan, Albert Starr, and later, Andrius Grüntzig, and many others, whom he came to respect greatly. [17] Yet he was sometimes unpredictable as a panelist. He unhesitatingly interrupted another speaker if he disagreed with him and berated him. Although audiences grew to expect these diatribes, some squirmed in their seats. Sones was always the patients' advocate. He was particularly critical of randomized studies. In later years, convinced of the benefit of bypass graft surgery, he blasted attempts by the more scientifically minded to organize a randomized trial of bypass surgery, comparing it to the notorious Tuskegee Syphilis trial in which black prisoners with syphilis were randomized to either placebo, or to antibiotic treatment.

Sones was well known for his verbal abuse of "authorities" who spread misinformation advertised as fact at medical meetings. A young physician was presenting at the American Heart Association a paper on myocardial infarction in the absence of coronary artery disease. There were two cases and the coronary arteriogram of one was shown—probably the better film. The young speaker seemed modest and Mason liked him. The patients had been studied in the laboratory at Peter Bent Brigham Hospital. A co-author of the paper was Richard Gorlin, a friend of Mason. After the presentation, the discussion was opened by Mason Sones. He said, "I would like to point out that the arteriogram showed total occlusion of the anterior descending artery." The silence was deafening. After a short pause the young investigator said, "I bow to the master of coronary arteriography and apologize for presenting this report."

Several months later the same young man visited Sones in the laboratory for a week. Mason treated him with the same respect that he displayed for distinguished cardiologists.

On another occasion Dr. William Likoff, a well-known cardiologist from Hahnemann Medical School, gave a presentation on angina with normal coronary arteries. He illustrated his talk with a rather poor quality cineangiogram that included a left ventriculogram, which showed systolic anterior motion of the anterior mitral valve leaflet, a phenomenon, then unreported, characteristic of idiopathic hypertrophic subaortic stenosis (then known as muscular subaortic stenosis or myocardial dysplasia). Sones and colleagues were aware of this association, and Sones verbally blasted Likoff for not recognizing the obvious—that there was another explanation for the patient's chest pain. (At the same meeting Sones talked on coronary arteriography and showed a left ventriculogram that he considered to be normal, but later came to be recognized as typical of mitral valve prolapse.) Although Sones and colleagues had observed many new angiographic phenomena they never reported them in the medical literature. Sones was never interested in credit for a new observation.

On still another occasion, during a talk Sones was strongly critical of Arthur Vineberg who had introduced the internal mammary artery implant procedure. Vineberg was in the audience. Later he learned that Vineberg's wife was also with him, and Sones was deeply chagrined that he had embarrassed Vineberg in the presence of his family.

One day in 1968 Sones was studying a patient with Robert Quint, a fellow, assisting. With the Philips Co. he had devised a rotating cradle for the tabletop that facilitated rotating the patient into different projections for optimal angiographic views. This necessitated a mounting for the image amplifier that allowed it to be rotated aside when the patient was placed on the cradle. The patient developed ventricular fibrillation after an injection into one of his coronary arteries. As instructed to facilitate closed chest massage and defibrillation, the nurse swung the image amplifier aside, and in doing so it struck

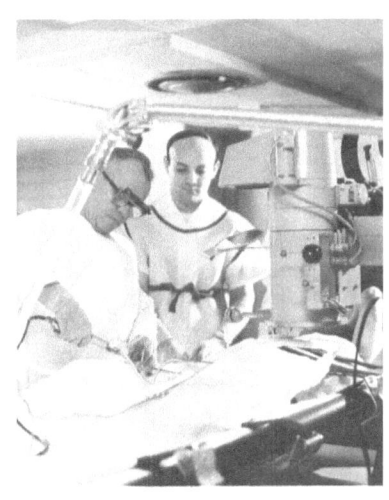

Sones and Robert A. Quint

Quint on the head, knocking him to the floor, briefly unconscious. When Sones called for the defibrillator paddles Quint was unable to respond. Looking around Sones saw Quint on the floor and in a rage said, "Get up off your lazy ass, Quint, and get me those fucking paddles!" Quint did respond, the patient was successfully defibrillated, and Quint had no recollection of the episode. A small abrasion on his head documented the event.

Sones spent little time with his family, Gerry his wife, or his children: sons Mason Jr., Steven and David, and daughter Patty. The lifestyle took its toll, however, and in 1963 Gerry filed for divorce. This made things only worse for him and he became more irascible and short tempered. He was working later, drinking more, and arriving later in the lab after a late night at the Theatrical Grill.

From the 1960s through the 1980s the Theatrical Grill was a favorite watering hole for Cleveland businessmen, lawyers and a few Clinic physicians. Mushy Wechsler, an ex-felon, was the owner. It was noted for its outstanding food and jazz bands. Sones regularly went there after work, often with visitors. On one occasion after an evening at the Theatrical, he awakened the following morning to discover that his car was missing from its usual spot in the garage, and then recalled arriving home in a taxi the previous night. Certain that his car had been stolen, he filed a stolen vehicle report with the police, and took a taxi to work at the Clinic. That evening he went to the Theatrical Grill as usual, and fumed at Mushy and his lousy security for having allowed his car to be stolen. Mushy smiled and took him to a parking lot across the street and found his car where he had parked it the evening before. Mushy explained that Sones was in no condition to drive the previous night, and sent him home in a taxi. He never again complained about Mushy's security. [18]

Irvine Page described Sones well:

> All those who know Sones have great respect for him, especially for three qualities—his unflinching demand for technical excellence, his courage, and his creativity. A tireless worker, he demands as much of those training under him, who now constitute a large international group. His volatile temperament and his frankness can be disconcerting, but those of us who know him recognize this is merely a spillover of his born enthusiasm and boundless drive. The timid and lazy find him a trial; the active and dedicated, an inspiration.

By 1965, when he succeeded Ernstene as Department Chairman, Proudfit had developed a busy clinical practice, to which most of Ernstene's patients were added. By now he had become known as a brilliant clinician and teacher. Royston Lewis had been appointed to the staff in 1962, and the Department of Clinical Cardiology consisted of Westcott, Royston Lewis, and himself. Clinical Cardiology and the Department of Cardiovascular Disease and the Cardiac Laboratory each had separate training programs for fellows. Fellows from Proudfit's department observed cath procedures in the cardiac laboratory, and those from Sones' Department rotated through the ECG laboratory to learn ECG interpretation, a not entirely satisfactory system.

In 1965, constrained by the confines of the surgical Pavilion on the second floor of the Hospital, under pressure from Effler and his colleagues, the Board of Governors shut down the obstetrical department on the sixth floor of the hospital to make way for three new cardiac operating rooms and a post-surgical intensive care unit.

44

C. Charles Welch joined Clinical Cardiology in 1965. A graduate of Northwestern University, he did his internship, internal medicine residency and cardiology training in the U.S. Navy in Oakland, Great Lakes, and Bethesda.

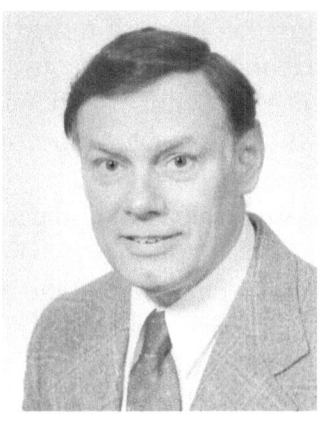

In 1966 James R. Hodgman, a graduate of the University of Michigan and a fellow in Internal Medicine and Cardiovascular Disease at the Clinic, became the fifth member of Clinical Cardiology.

James R. Hodgman

With increasing referrals for valve surgery Shirey developed a method for assessing mitral stenosis with retrograde catheterization of the left atrium—across the aortic and mitral valves. He developed a special long tapered catheter that facilitated this approach.[15]

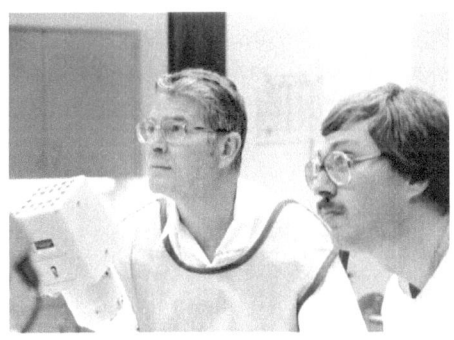

Earl K. Shirey and Fellow

Shirey had also become interested in needle biopsy of the left ventricle In 1967 Likoff presented a report of fifteen premenopausal women with angina and normal coronary arteriograms. He concluded that they had microvascular disease that could not be identified by coronary arteriography, and this was called "Syndrome X."[16] Shirey performed transthoracic myocardial biopsies of the left ventricle on 39 patients who underwent coronary arteriography for suspected coronary artery disease, with and without demonstrable disease. Three of 16 patients with severe coronary atherosclerosis had small vessel disease with fibrosis and thickening of the media. These patients clinically, in addition to chest pain, had congestive failure and/or recurrent ventricular tachycardia. None of the patients with normal coronary arteriograms had small vessel disease on biopsy. By 1972 his myocardial biopsy experience was among the world's largest, more than 300 patients, and he became the local expert in primary myocardial disease.[17,18]

In 1966 Proudfit turned over the directorship of the electrocardiography laboratory to Westcott but continued to share the reading responsibility. The ECG Laboratory now consisted of a Hospital section and the Desk 81 section where most of the ECG reading occurred.

Also in 1966 Proudfit published the first in a series of studies correlating the coronary arteriogram with clinical findings in 1000 patients. This landmark work demonstrated the pitfalls of clinical diagnosis. Only *typical* angina pectoris, or clinical and electrocardiographic signs of myocardial infarction reliably identified severe coronary disease with 90 percent confidence. This was the first in a series of articles correlating clinical characteristics with angiographic findings in various subsets of patients.[19-22]

After fifteen months at home in Argentina which he found unsympathetic to new concepts in cardiac surgery, Rene Favaloro returned in December 1966 to join Effler and Groves in Cardiac Surgery. By now he was an expert surgeon, skilled in valve replacements, internal mammary implantation and coronary endarterectomy. Working with Effler he helped develop modifications of the internal mammary implant operation, and he invented a chest retractor that facilitated mobilization of both internal mammary arteries for implantation.

Coronary Artery Bypass Graft Surgery

On May 3, 1967 Dr. Eugene Biagioni, a fellow working under the supervision of David Fergusson studied a 57 year old woman with class ii-iii angina. The right coronary artery was completely obstructed in its midportion but retrograde filling by collaterals from the left coronary artery indicated the obliterated segment was quite short. The notes in the chart indicate that Drs. Fergusson and Biagioni envisioned that flow to the right coronary artery could be reconstituted with a right internal mammary artery anastomosis to the distal right coronary artery. Dr. Favaloro was consulted and she was accepted for surgery. On May 9, 1967 Favaloro performed an interposition saphenous vein graft between the proximal and distal segments of the right coronary artery. It was never clear why Favaloro chose to do a vein graft instead of an internal mammary artery anastomosis. Fergusson and Biagioni performed a followup angiogram two weeks after surgery and confirmed patency of the graft and normal flow through the right coronary system. Although bypass graft operations had been performed by others, (and by Favaloro in September 1967), none of the previous operations was thought to have been successful and none had been reported in the surgical literature.[23-25] [19] This event revolutionized the surgical treatment of coronary artery disease. A few days after studying Favaloro's first patient a very excited Sones took the cine with him on a trip to Europe and the word was out. Favaloro published his experience with 15 cases—including one aortocoronary bypass—in 1968 (55 cases by the time of publication).[26]

New Surgical Vistas

In 1968, after Christiaan Barnard's first cardiac transplant operation of December 2, 1967 [20], the Clinic team of Effler, Groves and Favaloro performed two cardiac transplants: the first survived two years, then died suddenly; the second died in one month of acute rejection. At this point Effler called a halt to further transplant procedures until the rejection issues could be resolved. In 1968 Favaloro began performing bypass surgery on patients with impending or acute myocardial infarction with encouraging results.[27] Favaloro also performed internal mammary to coronary artery grafts on two patients in 1970. The internal mammary artery graft to native coronary arteries had been popularized by Dr. George Green of New York.[28] Favaloro found the optical assistance that Green advocated too cumbersome to be practical and abandoned the technic.

The Judkins Approach

Charles Dotter, a radiologist at the University of Oregon, had learned a percutaneous technic of catheterizing the femoral artery from Sven-Ivar Seldinger of the Karolinska Institute in Stockholm. In 1964 he recanalized the femoral artery of an 83 year old woman with the combination of a guide wire and a catheter. Melvin Judkins, a radiologist also at the University of Oregon, began using the Seldinger technic that he had learned from Dotter in angiographic studies. In November 1967 he published a paper describing an alternative approach to coronary arteriography, a percutaneous method from the right femoral artery with specially designed preformed catheters, and with cut-film rather than motion picture (cine) photography.[29] Sones and colleagues were skeptical of this approach, in which skin resistance at the entry point reduced the operator's tactile sensitivity for guiding the catheter that was afforded by the brachial approach. Nevertheless, by avoiding a surgical cutdown the method rapidly gained popularity. Several instances were observed of catheter dissections of coronary arteries due to the sharp-edged end-hole of the extruded Judkins catheter, but Judkins was quick to point out the potential risks and means of avoiding complications. After he had accomplished 100 studies Judkins called Sones in 1967 and invited him to visit his laboratory. Sones was cool and replied that this was an insufficient experience to evaluate the technique and to call him again after he had done 600 cases as Sones had done. Judkins did just that, and when Sones visited his laboratory a few months later he was impressed that Judkins was not only highly skilled and knowledgeable, but his angiograms—cut films, not cines—were of excellent quality and he shared Sones' commitment to safety of the procedure. Ultimately these rivals from different disciplines, Sones a cardiologist and Judkins a radiologist, became close friends and highly respectful of each other. In 1978 they joined forces to co-found the Society for Cardiac Angiography, a guild of experts dedicated to the achievement of the highest quality and safety in the performance of cardiac angiography.

In 1968 there was growing unrest with the Clinic's governance. The medical staff now numbered in the hundreds. Hospital beds were again filled to capacity despite the addition of a new southwest wing in the mid 1960s. Although the Board of Governors was responsible for the professional side of Clinic management, including appointments to the Staff and medical policies, they had little influence over the business management and the hospital. This was the responsibility of the Trustees, through a business manager, and a hospital administrator both of whom reported directly to the Trustees who followed a particularly conservative fiscal policy. The Clinic had assiduously avoided any long-term debt since the 1929 fire. The Trustees did not believe that physicians could manage the financial aspects of the enterprise. The medical staff was growing restless and became disenchanted with the administration. Capital needs were not being met to sustain a bourgeoning practice.

Proudfit, Effler and Sones were particularly unhappy. The Business Manager had informed Sones that because of budgetary constraints a replacement X-ray tube would have to be purchased with Department funds earmarked for research and education. There were growing referrals for coronary arteriography and cardiac surgery. The first coronary bypass operation had been performed in 1967, and although the long term benefit of this procedure was as yet unclear, it did seem to be promising. Frustrated, Sones accepted an invitation to meet with Dr. Michael DeBakey at Methodist Hospital in Houston to discuss the possibility of moving there. Methodist Hospital had just constructed a new facility in which there was a generous amount of space available for new cardiac laboratories. At the moment this seemed to be his only alternative and he discussed the proposition with Shirey and Sheldon suggesting that they join him in the move to Houston. Reluctantly we agreed to consider the possibility. He returned to Houston for a second round of discussions, this time proposing that Effler be included in the move. DeBakey demurred, and the move was never discussed again. Sones and Effler badgered Clinic's leaders for new facilities.

New Governance

In the summer of 1968 a small delegation from the medical staff met secretly with some of the Trustees at Cleveland's Union Club, the outcome of which would change the Clinic forever. The business manager was removed, and a new Business Manager and Hospital Administrator were appointed who would report to the Board of Governors, not the Trustees.

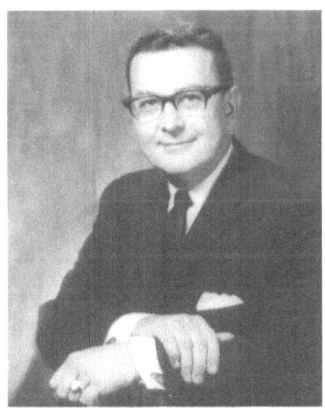

The Board of Governors was to manage the day-to-day administration of the Clinic and the Hospital, subject to oversight of the Trustees. LeFevre, who was highly respected by both the medical staff and Trustees, had served as Chairman of the Board of Governors for more than twelve years and was ready to step down; a search would be undertaken for his successor. A new business manager was appointed, [21] and the Hospital Administrator continued, both now reporting to the Board of Governors. The Trustees continued to be the authority responsible for all Clinic property,

Carl E. Wasmuth

overall fiscal policy, investments, and staff compensation. [22] A short time later on January 2, 1969, Dr. Carl Wasmuth, then Chairman of the Department of Anesthesiology and who also had a law degree, was elected by the Board to be its new Chairman. Some Trustees were still skeptical of this new arrangement.

In February 1969 Wasmuth presented to the Executive Committee of the Trustees a "white paper" that had previously been approved unanimously by the Board of Governors. This paper established the authority of the Board of Governors to assume the responsibility for operation of the entire Foundation. The Executive Committee approved the white paper. This was the "magna carta" of the Board of Governors.[30] (In this reorganization the Chairman the Division of Research, who previously had reported directly to the Trustees, now also reported to the Board of Governors. [23]) A short time later the new business manager and the hospital administrator resigned and were replaced by officers appointed by the Board of Governors. Wasmuth proved to be a prudent leader and the Clinic thrived.

One of Wasmuth's first acts was to appoint a long range planning committee.

Planning for a New Hospital and Clinic

The Long Range Planning Committee began to consider a new hospital wing, and an adjacent structure that would house the three cardiovascular departments in close proximity to their hospital functions, the operating rooms, intensive care units, and catheterization laboratories. Predictably this had a chilling effect upon other clinical departments who decried such blatant favoritism and a scheme that would geographically divide the Clinic. Moreover, bypass graft surgery had just begun and no one was certain what the future might bring. Nevertheless the decision was made in 1969 to proceed with a new hospital and outpatient facilities, even if it necessitated incurring debt. Later, as construction progressed, the Clinic was doing very well financially [24] and Wasmuth was optimistic that the new hospital and outpatient facilities might be paid for by current revenue and debt financing might not be necessary. That optimism proved to be unfounded however. (Construction of the Park Plaza Hotel, opposite the Clinic on East 96th Street began in 1972, and a new building to house the Research Division—the FF building—was completed in 1974).

Another early action by Wasmuth was to appoint a committee to explore the use of computers in clinical practice. A.W. Humphries was Chairman; Sheldon was one of the members. Several medical facilities had implemented computer applications, notably Latter Day Saints Hospital in Salt Lake City under Homer Warner, where patients in intensive care units were monitored comprehensively with computers. Humphries began a massive project, hired a large team of experts, and designed computerized workstations for the nursing floors in the new hospital addition. The Clinic had purchased a Honeywell computer that served several administrative functions, but no mainframe computer company could be found that would serve all the functions that Humphries envisioned. After considerable expense that project failed, but not before planting the seeds that would soon become the patient-doctor scheduling system and the hospital bed management system, and registries for cancer and cardiovascular data.

Proudfit was elected to the Board of Governors in 1969. This was a particularly critical time, as Wasmuth needed the strong support of the Board to carry out his agenda for restructuring and growth. One of the issues that came up was the question of allowing department and division chairmen to continue until the then mandatory retirement age of 65. Recent experience had raised this question when there were no obvious inside successors when a department chairman retired having reached 65, and an urgent outside search had to be undertaken. Some felt that if department heads and division chairmen would step down at age 60 this would allow a more orderly search and transition for their successors. Proudfit endorsed this concept, even recognizing that he might be one of the first to be affected—he would be 60 in 1974. The Board passed the resolution in 1970. Rupert Turnbull, Chairman of Colon and Rectal Surgery since 1968, became 60 in 1973 and was the first department head to be affected by the new policy. [25] The mandatory *retirement* age of 65 for all members of the professional staff continued, however, until the 1990's.

In the meanwhile several members of the staff had been having open discussions about a reorganization of the Clinic that would recognize disease-oriented groups of departments,—neurological, musculoskeletal, gastrointestinal—each becoming a division that would be represented on the Board of Governors, emulating the relationship that had evolved with the three cardiovascular departments, (although they had no permanent representative on the Board of Governors). [26]

The concept of disease-oriented divisions was doomed to failure however, because no one in a division of disease-related-departments could agree on who would be the division chairman. Nevertheless the discussions did promote closer cooperation between medical and surgical departments, i.e. Hypertension and Nephrology with Urology, Rheumatology with Orthopedic Surgery, Gastroenterology with General Surgery and Colon and Rectal Surgery, Neurology with Neurosurgery etc.

Later, in 1969, Sones married Phyllis Kapell, whom he had met at the Bolton Square Hotel when her husband was recovering from heart surgery. After a brief courtship and her divorce, they were married, improbably, in Donald Effler's home. Phyllis had a beneficial effect on him. She insisted that he get home in time for them to have dinner together. He ate regularly, drank less, kept better hours, and again arrived at work at a more reasonable hour. At her insistence they regularly played golf together on Wednesday afternoons. She accompanied him on nearly all of his travels.

The Bruschke Era

Albert V.G. Bruschke, a young cardiologist from Utrecht, Netherlands first visited the Clinic in 1964 to learn coronary arteriography from Sones. Lacking ECFMG certification he could only be an observer. He spent several weeks watching procedures (with a periscope-mirror viewer on the image intensifier) and, like Favaloro, he devoured everything he could about coronary arteriography, reviewing hundreds of angiograms during the short time he was there. When he returned to Utrecht he was the first in the Netherlands, and possibly in all Europe, to perform the procedure. He

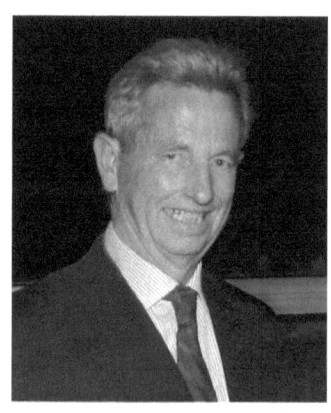

Albert V.G. Bruschke

returned periodically to the Clinic, and with the evolution of coronary artery surgery, began to consider the potential value of assessing the clinical course of patients based upon their coronary artery anatomy. Effler had already pronounced severe left main and proximal anterior descending lesions as "widow-makers."

In 1970 when Sones was on a lecture tour in Europe Bruschke met him again. He mentioned his interest in doing a followup study of patients whose coronary disease was documented by coronary arteriography. Sones and Proudfit had discussed a similar endeavor, as an extension of

Proudfit's correlative studies of clinical characteristics of patients as related to coronary anatomy. Sones interest was piqued and he hired Bruschke on the spot. When Bruschke returned to the Clinic in 1970 Sones arranged for him to be appointed a special fellow, and informed an unsuspecting Proudfit that he was to supervise the project. Sones had already recused himself from participating in any correlative analyses because he thought nobody would believe him. Bruschke had not met Proudfit until then, but Proudfit befriended him and there began a memorable friendship and productive collaboration.

Proudfit writes:[9]

> On July 1, Albert appeared in my office and I took him to the Education Building. I explained that we would like him to collect two series of patients: one group with normal or almost normal coronary arteries and the other with significant disease (a minimum of 50 percent narrowing of a major artery or a principal branch). Consecutive cases were to be used, eliminating only those known to have had an operation for coronary disease within two years of catheterization. Patients with valvular heart disease, hypertensive heart disease and subaortic stenosis, or primary myocardial disease were also excluded. Many of these patients had no follow-up after discharge following cardiac catheterization. All patients were eligible to have survived for a minimum of 5 years. I explained that we had only the code sheets that I had used for our correlative studies of clinical and arteriographic findings. These must be modified. Some of the coding was to be done without knowledge of catheterization findings. Albert could have bowed out in view of our unpreparedness but he accepted the assignment without blinking. A week later Albert appeared in my office with tentative code sheets, some follow-up letters, and plans for follow-up. I could hardly believe that he had accomplished so much. He planned to mail letters to the referring physicians and then write to patients after two weeks if he had no response. A second letter to the patient might be sent. Failure of written response required telephone inquiry. He soon discovered that Americans are mobile and may be difficult to trace, especially after a lapse of some years.

This preliminary work was followed by a period of intense activity, selecting the two study groups and mailing letters. He had 521 in the normal group and 620 in the abnormal. Piles of mail appeared daily and Bruschke read all the responses immediately. If further information was required, he telephoned the referring physician, the local hospital, or the patient. Albert had a background in statistics, so he realized that follow-up should be as complete as possible. He developed some ingenious original methods of follow-up and ultimately followed 500 of 521 in the normal group and 590 of the 620 (95%) abnormals. Later in doing a 10 year survival study of the abnormal group, several college girls were able to achieve 100 percent follow-up of the abnormal group. Following the additional 30 patients did not alter the conclusions significantly. Albert's original 95% 5-9 year follow-up of the abnormal group was considered remarkable at that time.

In May 1971, Albert completed his studies and wrote drafts of the manuscripts of three papers: the prognosis in the normal or almost normal group, the prognosis in relation to arteriographic findings in the abnormal group, and the prognosis in relation to ventriculographic findings. Only Mason's approval was required for submission for publication. Bruschke decided to write abstracts for presentation of the three studies of the fall meeting of the American Heart Association. Mason approved. At that time the majority of abstracts were accepted for printing in the abstract book, so Bruschke and I were annoyed when only the abstract of the normal group was accepted for publication and the other two abstracts were rejected. Sones was not surprised, in fact he seemed rather pleased that the selection committee was so resistant to progress. Although Bruschke polished his manuscripts a bit during June while waiting for Sones to read them and approve for submission to the editor of *Circulation,* we could not get Sones to read them. He did get Bruschke's fellowship extended two months and Albert continued to make minor changes in his manuscripts. Each day I asked Mason if he had read the texts, and he promised that he would do so "tonight" or "tomorrow." By late August, Albert was getting desperate, because he had tickets to return to Holland and his teaching position. Finally

Mason said he would review the manuscripts with us "tonight" (about August 27). We met in his office and it was evident that he had not read any of the manuscripts. However, Albert patiently explained each text to him and we were astonished at the rapidity of his grasp. It was a long evening and Sones had a few suggestions that required a little review of original data. One point, however, would necessitate extensive search of the data. Bruschke agreed that Sones had a valid objection. I feared that Albert would be discouraged and give up. I said that I would do the search and send him the results, so that all of the manuscripts could be revised slightly. Albert said that the responsibility was his, and he worked night and day for three days. After about two weeks I received the corrected copies and submitted the three manuscripts to Dr. Howard Burchell, Editor of *Circulation*. A few days later I had a call from Howard, saying that these were three classic papers that would be published in *Circulation*. He added that he would not ask for peer review—a most unusual action. I told him that abstracts of two of the studies had been rejected by the selection committee of the American Heart Association for the fall meeting. He laughed and said, "That tells you something about committees." Mason was pleased and seemed to be unaware that he had inconvenienced Albert. Bruschke was delighted and showed no rancor toward Mason.

It was this database that facilitated no fewer than six original papers on the natural history of patients with and without coronary artery disease, the first of which appeared in 1973. Many of these are still currently cited.[31-36]

Coronary Intensive Care

Although Proudfit and Sones first suggested that the Clinic create a coronary constant care unit in 1965, it was not until 1970 that an area on the fourth floor of the old hospital (4-East) was remodeled as a coronary intensive care unit with Royston Lewis as its first Director. The new coronary intensive care unit had four beds, and a large room equipped as a cardiac catheterization laboratory. Sones envisioned one day performing coronary arteriograms routinely in patients with acute myocardial infarction. Although never used for that purpose, the room was used for insertion of temporary pacemakers, and ultimately it became the first pacemaker laboratory under Lon Castle. (Hodgman succeeded Lewis as Director of the CICU in 1972).

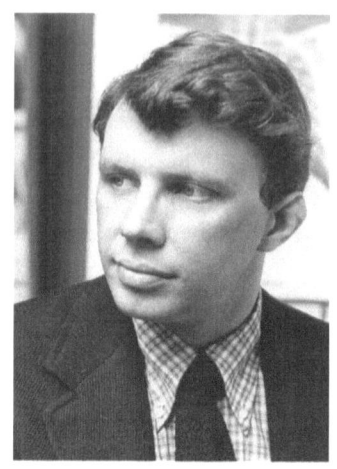

Floyd D. Loop

Floyd D. Loop and Chalit Cheanvechai both completed their fellowships in Cardiac Surgery at the Clinic in 1970 and joined Effler, Groves and Favaloro in the Department of Thoracic and Cardiac Surgery. Both were quickly recognized for their technical skills as well as their personal qualities. Sones befriended both, and soon would refer his surgical cases only to them. As Loop began to travel more frequently, Cheanvechai became Sones' main surgical consultant, and operated on virtually all of his patients. At one point Sones entered the minefield of surgical staff compensation and tried to persuade Effler to increase Cheanvechai's salary. Whether he succeeded will never be known but the effort did little for the Effler-Sones relationship. One of the Clinic's busiest cardiac surgeons, Cheanvechai returned to practice in his native Thailand shortly after Loop replaced Effler as Department Head in 1975.

Internal Mammary Artery Grafts

In January 1971 Loop began to perform left internal mammary (thoracic) artery anastomoses to the anterior descending. [27] Early postoperative studies showed a patency in excess of 95%. Subsequent studies showed an attrition rate that was far less than for venous grafts, and the superiority of IMA grafts was evident by 1972.[37,38]

In March 1972 Joel Webster and Carl Moberg, a fellow in Sones' Department, presented to the annual scientific session of the American College of Cardiology their followup study of 526 patients with severe proximal coronary artery constructions studied between 1960 and 1965, who did not have any surgical revascularization procedure. This was one of the first "natural history" studies of patients with angiographically documented coronary artery disease. At the outset of their study the authors may not have been aware that Bruschke, under Proudfit's guidance, had initiated a similar study of patients from the years 1963-1965. Although Webster included Sones' name as an author of the presentation,[39] Sones, of course, was aware of the Proudfit-Bruschke effort and he objected strenuously to Webster's paper. After its presentation, Webster had submitted the paper to the *American Journal of Cardiology* for publication. Sones demanded that the paper be rescinded. When Webster refused, Sones called the editor of AJC to block the publication. Although the editor refused to interfere, the paper was not published until 1974, by authors Webster, Moberg and Rincon.[40] Webster left the Clinic for private practice in Charlotte, North Carolina in 1973. Bruschke and Proudfit published the first papers on their followup studies in 1973.

In the meanwhile Sheldon had analyzed results of coronary endarterectomy and early vein graft operations, and presented this work at the AHA in 1968.[41] He began a followup study of the first 1000 patients with vein graft surgery, operated upon between 1967 and 1970. This was presented at the annual meeting of the American Heart Association in November 1972 and published in *Circulation* the following year.[42] Although some of these patients had associated revascularization procedures, and Webster and Moberg's nonsurgical patients were used for comparison, a non-contemporaneous group with severe proximal coronary obstructions, this study suggested that surgical treatment improved the survival of patients with more severe disease, i.e. left main coronary disease and triple vessel disease, and least beneficial for patients with single vessel disease. Later the study was refined to include only patients with vein graft surgery, and the findings were the same.[43] The conclusions were essentially confirmed by later multicenter randomized studies.

Wayne Siegel went to medical School at The University of Miami School of Medicine and did summer medical student fellowships at the Scripps Clinic in La Jolla, and at the National Childrens Cardiac Hospital in Miami. After completing an Internal Medicine residency at the Clinic he joined the U.S. Public Health Service and worked at Southwestern University Medical School in Dallas where he worked in exercise physiology and worked with computer systems and ultrasound transducers in the research laboratory. Subsequently he furthered his interest in echocardiography as a NIH Research Fellow at Emory University. He joined Proudfit's Department in 1971 where he started an echocardiography laboratory and performed bicycle ergometer stress tests in two small rooms on the fifth floor of the hospital.

In the same year Frederick Heupler, a graduate of the University of Pennsylvania, completed his fellowship in Cardiovascular Disease at the Clinic and joined Sones' Department. Both Siegel and Heupler were excellent clinicians and astute observers. Siegel recalled one patient with whom they collaborated in documenting coronary artery spasm:[44]

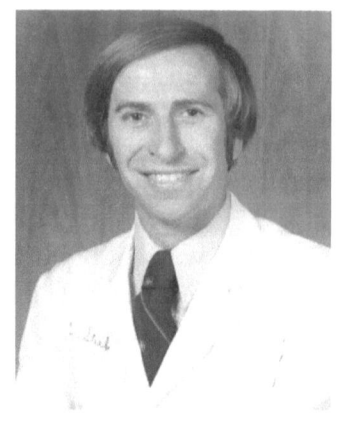

Wayne Siegel

It was about 1974 when a psychiatric n u r s e   f r o m Michigan was sent to me for functional testing. She was having angina pectoris at rest as well as at times provoked by exertion or emotional stress. Her stress test, echo and physical exam were completely normal. Fred Heupler did a diagnostic cath for me and this too was normal. When I gave her report to her something felt amiss. She was certain that something was wrong and because of that occasional moment of transference that we may have with patients, I felt that in fact she was right . . . . something was wrong. I put her to bed in the CCU.

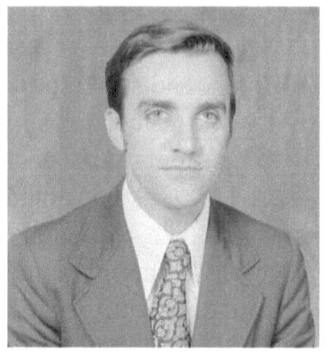

Frederick Heupler

The next day I was on rounds and after seeing the rest of my patients, I went to the CCU and stayed with her. I remember standing at the foot of her bed just chatting with her when she got this horrific look on her face and then she blurted, "I am starting to have an attack!" I looked at her monitor and felt a very strong and very real feeling of absolute panic as her ST segments began to elevate and elevate and elevate. She literally writhed in pain. I turned on the recorder as she went into ventricular bigeminy and then intermittent complete heart block. I gave her a nitro. In moments the pain abated, the rhythm returned to sinus and the ST segments normalized. It was as though God or serendipity or whatever Karma there is in this universe had placed this woman at my service. I called Bill Proudfit.

That day we reviewed her angios with Fred and then Earl. They were normal. Bill and Roy had previously tried Ergot in the 1960s as a bedside test for angina. It was too dangerous for patients with anatomical obstructions so they discontinued their trials. I believe there was something about a myocardial infarction, but I am not sure of that. I knew of the power of Nitroprusside from Harriet Dustan's work and I suggested that we do an ergonovine infusion on my patient with nitroprusside ready to go as an antidote. Bill and the patient agreed and so we brought her into the Cardiac Function Lab. and sure enough "BINGO" we provoked the whole thing and reversed it immediately. It was then that I decided to ask Fred to repeat her cath and allow me to repeat my ergonovine-nitroprusside salvo. He agreed.

The next day, Bill Proudfit, Fred Heupler and yours truly marched down that wonderful lane of de novo clinical research with a very trusting patient. To this day I have never seen anyone do a more rapid and complete coronary angiogram than Fred did that day after we infused Ergonovine and provoked TOTAL proximal obstruction of the right coronary artery! He was a blur. And we had documented angiographically for the first time that functional coronary spastic disease was real and potentially lethal.

In a short time Mason Sones called me into his office and forcefully told me that if I ever published this information I would be fired. I went to Fred and told him that this study and those to follow would have to be carried out by the cath lab group and that I wanted Fred to carry the ball. I was clearly intimidated and quite upset about Mason's personal threat. Irrational, yes, but real!

In time we submitted an abstract to AHA and Fred presented the beginning of his series.[45]

By 1971 patient referrals to the three cardiovascular departments were soaring, and became almost unmanageable. Despite five catheterization laboratories in the basement (B-10), and three operating rooms on the sixth floor of the hospital (opened in 1970 in space vacated by the closure of the Department of Obstetrics), waiting lists for cardiac catheterization and cardiac surgery were growing longer. The Clinic Inn and the Hospital were full. Emergencies were difficult to accommodate and "pseudoemergencies" were becoming rampant. Angiograms of "mail order" patients who had their catheterization studies performed elsewhere were sent directly to the surgeons for review and surgical scheduling. These studies were, in turn, referred to members of Sones' department for review and opinion. Even these outside film reviews became backlogged.

The Tri Departmental Meetings

Members of the three departments mutually agreed to hold regular meetings to try to address these problems of a burgeoning referral practice. The first of these was held on Saturday February 20, 1971. Mehdi Razavi, who had joined the Staff in Sones' Department in 1967, served as Chairman and Recording Secretary. Occurring monthly on Saturday mornings, these sessions were enormously successful, if stressful. (After a few meetings Sones and Effler were quietly discouraged from attending—at least attending the same meetings together). Many issues were discussed that were unsettled if not controversial in contemporary cardiovascular care: the use of quinidine in the postoperative patient (Effler had banned its use after a spate of sudden deaths in patients treated with quinidine for postoperative atrial fibrillation); the question of anticoagulants in valve replacement patients—(anticoagulants were not routinely used after valve replacement surgery at the Clinic or at other centers and most patients seemed to do quite well. Each new valve prosthesis was deemed "safer" than its predecessors, and it was several years before anticoagulant prophylaxis became the standard of care.) We questioned the need to discontinue beta blockers (propranolol) preoperatively which the anesthesiologists had mandated, and concluded this policy was unnecessary and unwise. After Effler halted Friday hospital transfers which often seemed to be for the convenience of the referring physician, we began also to examine direct hospital admissions and the hospital waiting list for "urgent" surgery, and what constituted truly urgent indications. We established policies for mail order surgeries, outside film reviews, referring patients with carotid bruits for evaluation prior to cardiac surgery, combined coronary bypass/carotid endarterectomy procedures, postoperative cardioversions and many others related to patient selection and perioperative management.

The Cardiovascular Information Registry (CVIR)

At one of these meetings, in October 1971, Sheldon brought up the need for a computerized cardiovascular information management system. [28] Proudfit, Fergusson, Sheldon and Loop had all experienced the tribulations of chart reviews to record clinical data and conducting followup studies with IBM Hollerith cards, and computer technology was now available. A group consisting of Sheldon, Floyd Loop and Wayne Siegel agreed to study the feasibility of such a project. At the next Tri-Departmental meeting, on December 4, 1971, a definitive proposal was approved. Proudfit was added to the committee, and these four physicians set about developing the Cardiovascular Information Registry (CVIR), creating code sheets, recruiting support personnel, and identifying space and equipment needs. The three department chairmen agreed to assist with financial, space and equipment resources. Emily Wagstaff RN, a surgical nurse and research assistant in Cardiothoracic Surgery, was recruited to supervise the coding and data entry. Barry Rubinson, Dr. Siegel's computer technician for echocardiography, helped with the computer programming. By the end of 1972 all catheterization and surgical patients of that year were coded and ready for uploading into the Clinic's Honeywell mainframe computer. Later, all catheterization and surgical patients from 1967 through 1971 were added to the Registry, and complete data were now available on all coronary bypass patients. Data on valve surgery, thoracic aneurysms and surgical procedures for arrhythmias have been added in more recent years. This Registry continues today and is not only the largest, but it is the longest continuous cardiovascular registry of its kind. The CVIR is the key to monitoring quality and performance. It is the major resource for clinical cardiovascular research for all three departments, and has facilitated the regular reporting of cath lab complications, surgical experience, and follow-up studies of patients after cardiac surgery. [29]

The Tri-Departmental Meetings continued through the 1980s. Royston Lewis took over as Chairman and Recording Secretary in March 1974, and later, James Hodgman chaired the meetings (1976-1980). These meetings, in a sense, codified the relationship that had evolved between Cardiology and Cardiac Surgery since the early 1960s, and for the first time included Cardiothoracic Anesthesiology. In later years this relationship would be defined as an integrated practice unit, and contributed substantially to the continuing success of the Clinic's cardiovascular program.

This forum, however, fell into disuse in the 1980s after coronary angioplasty was introduced. Although we had achieved a consensus on the indications for surgical backup for interventional procedures, the interventional cardiologists soon began to accept sicker patients with unstable angina, acute myocardial infarction, hypotension and cardiac failure. When complications occurred in these patients our surgical colleagues grew weary and began to use these forums as an attempt to limit cath lab procedures. In later years, with improved interventional technology, and better patient selection, procedural risks diminished, emergency surgical referrals for complications of PCI declined, and bruised sensitivities were somewhat healed.

A Visit from Royalty

In early 1972 Crown Prince Khaled of Saudi Arabia was referred to the Clinic. He had sustained a myocardial infarction and was seen in consultation by Dr. Walter Sommerville of London. A postinfarction ventricular aneurysm was suspected and Sommerville suggested he come to the Clinic. With his entourage of hundreds he took over the Clinic Inn (which had recently been constructed on Carnegie and E. 91st St., replacing the old Bolton Square Hotel). Sones confirmed the diagnosis and Effler was to excise the aneurysm. Effler suggested to Sones that Mehdi Razavi, with his Persian background, be assigned to cover the medical care of the Crown Prince during his hospitalization. The surgery, in January 1972, was uneventful and the Crown Prince remained at the Clinic for about a month. All expected a generous contribution to the Clinic, but after Sones sent him a bill for $1 million, no contribution was forthcoming. However Razavi's unique assignment launched a lucrative Saudi Arabian practice and what ultimately became a valuable relationship between the Clinic and Saudi Arabia. Khaled became King in 1975 after the assassination of King Faisal. A $500,000 contribution from Khaled in July 1975 helped launch the Clinic's international educational exchange program. [30] He returned for a second operation in 1978.

In 1972 Paul C. Taylor joined Effler, Groves and Loop in Thoracic and Cardiovascular Surgery. In 1973 Richard Westcott, Director of the Electrocardiography laboratory died of bronchogenic carcinoma and Royston Lewis replaced him as Director of Electrocardiography. James Hodgman became Director of the Coronary Intensive Care Unit.

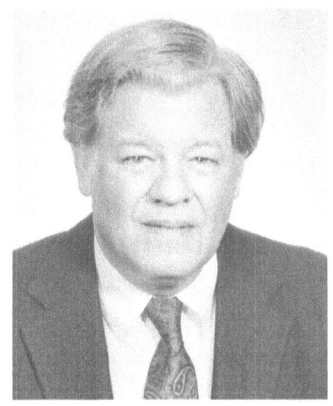

Paul C. Taylor

Further staff additions occurred in 1972 and 1973: Juan Lim (1972), Lon Castle (1973) and I.R. "Ravi" Rao (1973) in Clinical Cardiology, and Gustavo Rincon (1972), Augusto Pichard (1973), Hector Lardani (1973), and Daniel Phillips (1973) in the Department of Cardiovascular Disease and the Cardiac Laboratory. Lim was a graduate of Santo Tomas University in the Philippines and an internal medicine training program at St. Elizabeth Hospital in Youngstown, and cardiology fellowships at the Clinic and also at St. Michael Hospital in Toronto. Rao was also a Fellow in Cardiovascular Disease at the Clinic.

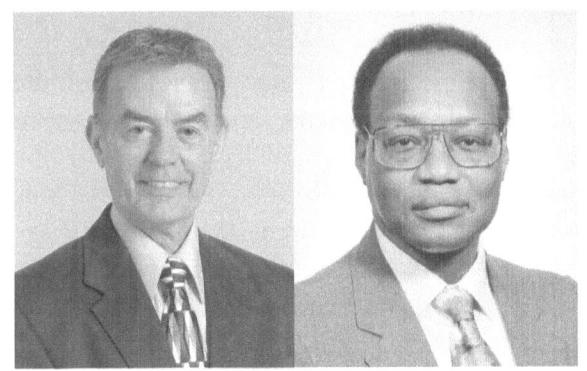

Lon A. Castle   Victor G. Morant

Lon Castle, a Temple University graduate, completed a fellowship in Cardiology at the Clinic in 1973 and was also appointed to the Staff in Clinical Cardiology. Castle became interested in cardiac pacemakers, and after spending a few weeks with Dr. William Parsonnet at Beth Israel Hospital in Newark, New Jersey, he was appointed head of the Pacemaker Laboratory, then part of the Coronary Intensive Care Unit on 4-East. He was joined in 1976 by Victor Morant, a Panamanian by birth, who was a graduate of Northwestern University Medical School and the Clinic's fellowship in Clinical Cardiology. Together they built a large following of pacemaker patients, established a Pacemaker Clinic, and performed the first HIS—bundle electrograms. Morant later became Director of Ambulatory Electrocardiography (Holter Laboratory), and also Hospital Telemetry. Castle also served as Assistant Team Physician to the Cleveland Browns.

Rincon, Pichard, Lardani and Phillips were all graduates of the Clinic's fellowship in Cardiovascular Disease. Rincon was a graduate of the National University of Bogota, Columbia and residencies in internal medicine at Youngstown Hospital and Mount Sinai Hospital in Chicago. Pichard was a graduate of the Catholic University of Chile. Hector Lardani was a native of Argentina, and Daniel Phillips was a Yale graduate.

Charles Bost was appointed to Sones' Department in 1973 but soon departed to serve a military obligation and did not return. He was later killed in an automobile accident. Robert Quint left in 1971 for private practice in San Jose, CA. Charles Welch left in 1974 to join the Scott & White Clinic in Temple Texas.

Designing a Cardiovascular Center

As planning and construction of the new hospital and outpatient facilities progressed, Sones envisioned an outpatient diagnostic center where cardiology patients could have their chest X-rays, electrocardiograms, and blood drawn all in the same facility on the first floor. This required the cooperation of Radiology and Laboratory Medicine, and was a departure from the traditional system in which patients had to move from one department to another for these routine studies. This diagnostic center was to be in close proximity to the outpatient examining rooms and offices of the three departments. Six new catheterization laboratories would be in the hospital next to the Department of Cardiovascular Disease on the second floor, Clinical Cardiology next to the ECG laboratory in the diagnostic center on the first floor, and Cardiac Surgery was to be on the second floor not far from its operating rooms and intensive care unit. The hospital tower would rise above the cardiovascular offices, laboratories and operating rooms. Four of the six new catheterization laboratories would actually be 3-room suites with pre- and post-procedure rooms adjacent to each laboratory. Two of the laboratories were single procedure rooms.

Sones' office was to be adjacent to one of the procedure rooms. It was a revolutionary plan that proved to be highly efficient. During the planning an echocardiography laboratory was added adjacent to the diagnostic center, and one of the catheterization laboratories was earmarked as the pacemaker laboratory. [31] There was nothing like it in the world! [32]

The move-in process began in December 1973, and was completed by January 1974. Shortly thereafter Effler launched an anti-smoking campaign and determined to make the cardiology and cardiac surgery floors of the new hospital non-smoking floors. Sones, still a heavy smoker, objected. He felt this was not what patients wanted. Enlisting the help of Edmund Notebart, Co-Administrator of the hospital, Effler posted no-smoking signs on the seventh and eighth hospital floors. That night Sones personally removed the signs. Effler had them replaced the next day, and Sones removed them again in the evening. Understandably, the other hospital administrators and nursing staff that witnessed this saga found it quite amusing. Finally it was agreed that Effler could make the seventh floor—where surgical patients were located—nonsmoking, but smoking would be allowed on the eighth floor where cardiology patients were housed. It was not until the late 1980s that the entire hospital and all outpatient facilities were made nonsmoking areas. [33]

Transition

Proudfit, age 60 in February 1974, in keeping with the Board of Governors 1970 policy regarding division chairmen and department heads, that he helped craft, submitted his resignation as Chairman of Clinical Cardiology. In October a search committee was appointed to nominate his successor. Donald Effler who had been Chairman of Cardiothoracic Surgery since 1948 would be 60 in 1975. A short time later another search committee was appointed to identify his successor.

The Search Committee considered the possibility of amalgamating the two cardiology departments and keeping Sones as head, but he had already expressed his displeasure with some members of Proudfit's Department, and some felt that it would place Sones in an overly dominant position to be the only surviving member of the Effler-Sones-Proudfit triumvirate. Sones was unwilling to step down and pleaded his case before the Board, unsuccessfully.

On March 14, 1975 the Search Committee for Proudfit's successor recommended to the Board of Governors that the Departments of Clinical Cardiology and Cardiovascular Disease and the Cardiac Laboratory be amalgamated into a single Department of Cardiology with William Sheldon as its Chairman. Sones and Proudfit were both named Senior Physicians, to continue their active clinical practices until each attained the age of mandatory retirement. Both men subsequently supported Sheldon; indeed Sones, Proudfit, Shirey and Sheldon continued their warm friendship. [34]

A few weeks later, on the recommendation of the Search Committee for Effler's successor, the Board appointed Floyd D. Loop as Chairman of the Department of Cardiothoracic Surgery. Shortly thereafter Effler resigned and moved to Syracuse, New York where he established the cardiac surgery program at St. Joseph's Hospital. [35]

Proudfit continued as a Senior Physician in the department with his busy practice, reading electrocardiograms, mentoring his associates and the fellows. He continued his followup studies of medical and surgical patients. He also continued as a sought-after manuscript reviewer for several leading medical journals; his reviews were always meticulous, insightful, and complete—even to the accuracy of references. In addition he was able to explore his interest in the history of medicine. He spent several summer vacations in London, England where he perused medical libraries (including the Hunter Library) for original articles. He wrote a number of papers on the history of medicine and cardiology (John Hunter, John Fothergill, and William Heberden).[46-48]

After he retired in 1979 he remained active and busy as a Consultant on the Emeritus Staff in Cardiology in much the same capacity, teaching electrocardiography, mentoring fellows and continuing his own research, but without patient responsibility. He relinquished his consultancy in 1986 and continued his manuscript reviews and writing from home.

During his 39 years at the Clinic Proudfit helped foster an ethic of patient care that was to make the Clinic famous and contribute to its growth. He was an excellent internist and cardiologist, and an outstanding teacher; he particularly enjoyed teaching physical diagnosis. He became a role model for his colleagues, and for his fellows. He led by example. He was a superb observer and many of his clinical correlations are recorded in his bibliography. After Sones he was the second cardiologist to coauthor a paper with a cardiac surgeon. [36] He was not a politician, and never pursued positions of leadership in national organizations, or even at the Clinic. He never indulged in profanity. He had no enemies, and was respected by everyone. He rarely spoke unkindly of anyone, and if he didn't approve of someone, or what they had done, he simply kept it to himself. He became a devoted friend and counselor to many. On one occasion in the early 1960s he counseled this author that the ultimate satisfaction in life was to become expert in something—anything. Alas, that advice went unfulfilled. His friendships with Sones, Bruschke and Favaloro were deep and unique. He always had a marvelous sense of humor, and a keen intellect that allowed him to recall countless quotations, minutiae from medical history, name, places and clinic lore. Today, at age 93, little of this has been lost.

Favaloro returned to Argentina in June 1971 to the great disappointment of all, but he had strong feelings about returning home and building a thoracic and cardiovascular center dedicated to patient care, cardiovascular research, and training a new generation of Argentinian physicians and surgeons. Internationally renowned, he created the Favaloro Foundation, and the Institute of Cardiology and Cardiovascular Surgery in Buenos Aires. The Institute emulated the National Heart, Lung, and Blood Institute in the United States. He poured all of his energy and fortune into the Institute. His beloved wife Toni died in the early 1990's. In the late 1990's Argentina's economy deteriorated, and Favaloro's Institute faced enormous losses from defaulted payments by the government and other payors. He pleaded with the President of Argentina to resume payments, to no avail. Broken and destitute, he took is own life on July 29, 2000 at age 77. [37]

After Effler left the Clinic in 1975 he became chief of cardiac surgery at St. Joseph's Hospital in Syracuse, NY where he worked with Goffredo Gensini, a friend of Sones and one of the first to perform coronary arteriography outside of the Clinic. In addition, as a colorful and articulate speaker Effler became a popular consultant in medical malpractice litigation, always as a witness for the defense. He underwent knee replacement surgery at the Clinic in the 1980s, and later a coronary angioplasty at St. Joseph's Hospital. He retired from practice in 1985 in failing health and died at age 89 in 2004.

Sones continued to do catheterizations in the new facilities he had designed. His office was a large room on the second floor overlooking the entrance to the hospital, adjacent to the catheterization laboratories. His window drapes were always drawn however, as he was always reviewing angiograms—those of his own patients, those brought for consultation by his colleagues, and those referred by hundreds of cardiologists around he world. He continued to travel extensively on speaking engagements. In 1978 he and Melvin Judkins co-founded the Society for Cardiac Angiography. In 1981 he was found to have a pulmonary nodule that was proved to be malignant. On resection it appeared to be well encapsulated and all were encouraged that the prognosis was excellent. [38] He returned to his work and traveling. For the first time he began to take vacation trips with his second wife Phyllis. He began to contemplate retirement, and found a condominium in Florida that seemed like an ideal retirement home. His personal funds were limited however, and he asked Phyllis to share in the financing. When she declined their marriage soured, and they were divorced in 1982 or 1983.

Sones received many honors and awards during his lifetime including Golden Eagle Awards for Cinematography (1963, 1966, 1969), the American Medical Association Film Award (1966), the Modern Medicine Distinguished Achievement Award (1966), the Theodora and Susan Cumming Foundation Humanitarian Award (1966), the Haile Selassie Lecturer, Royal College of Physicians, (1966), the University of Maryland School of Medicine Alumnus of the Year Award (1969), the Radiological Society of North America Gold Medalist (1979), the Favaloro Foundation Gold Medal(1979), and the Gairdner Foundation International Award (1969). He received honorary degrees from Western Maryland College (1969), the Federal University of Rio de Janeiro (1969), the Federal University of La Plata, Argentina (1979) and the Medical Times Physician of Excellence Award (1981). In 1983 he received the Albert Lasker Clinic Research Award.

"The First Decade of Bypass Graft Surgery for Coronary Artery Disease" was celebrated at an International Symposium September 15-17, 1977, "A Generation of Coronary Arteriography" was celebrated at a second International Symposium October 18-20, 1979, and Sones was honored at a special symposium November 12, 1983. All were held in Cleveland. In 1984 the United States Catheter and Instrument Company presented Sones and Shirey with a Golden Catheter award, on the occasion of the 100,000[th] coronary angiogram, and a short time later Philips Medical Systems Inc. presented the Clinic a $1 million grant for the Sones Laboratories. Despite all his imperfections and idiosyncrasies, everyone who knew Sones, including Clinic leadership, understood his compassion and recognized his genius.

A recurrence of his lung cancer was diagnosed in 1984. [39] This time radiation therapy was advised and he elected to have this supervised by Dr. Antonio Antunez, a radiation oncologist friend, formerly at the Clinic but now at Cleveland's University Hospitals. By now Sones had remarried his first wife, Gerry, who cared for him for his remaining days.

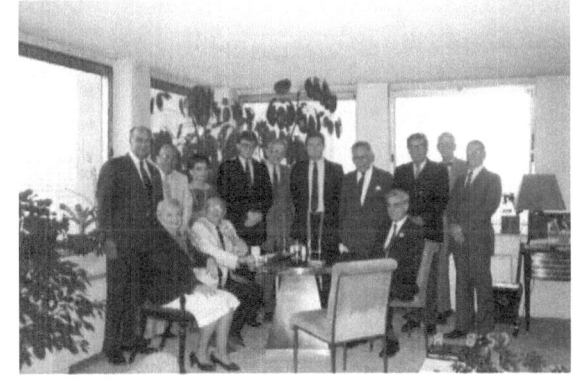

The Galen Medal Presentation

In 1985 he was to receive the Galen Medal of the historic Worshipful Society of Apothecaries of London, one of the oldest medical societies in the world. Sir Peter Tizard, Master of the Society wrote to Sones—twice, which Sones failed to answer. Weeks passed and he finally contacted Proudfit to intercede. [40] When it was explained that Sones was too ill to travel to London to receive the award, without precedent they agreed to present the award to him in his home in Cleveland. At a small but prestigious ceremony on July 27, 1985 attended by friends and colleagues, Sir Peter Tizard and the British Consul presented the award.

During his final weeks visits from dozens of friends and colleagues from around the world filled his days. Effler, too, wanted to pay is respects, convey his gratitude and express his friendship, but Sones demurred. He died quietly at home on August 29, 1985.

Notes to The Proudfit-Sones Years

1. Initially he did a few cases from the umbilical vein.
2. Shirey quotes Sones that Zimmerman's first case, performed from the left ulnar artery, and resulted in death. The catheter, believed to be in the left ventricle, was wedged in the left coronary artery. Cournand learned of this and strongly discouraged left heart catheterization studies. Andre Cournand, a respected cardiologist and early user of Forsmann's discovery, taught that catheterization of the left side of the heart was too hazardous for clinical application.
3. Sones later concluded that the 11-inch image amplifier was one of his greatest mistakes. Its large field size encompassed almost the entire chest of an adult, and an entire body of an infant, and had the effect of "minifying" the coronary arteries on 35 mm film. He later found that a five-inch amplifier was best for displaying coronary arteries and valves, and cardiac structures in infants.
4. Sones variously reported this as "20-30 ml," "approximately 30 ml," "40 ml" or "almost all of 50 ml;" "at least 30 cc" is what he described in the catheterization report. In the 1959 abstract he did not admit to direct intracoronary injections, only "20 to 30 ml into the right and left sinuses of Valsalva adjacent to the orifices of the vessels."[4]
5. Sones never benefited financially from these associations. In fact he assiduously avoided any ties with industry. On one occasion he had been invited to Albuquerque, New Mexico for the dedication of a new catheterization laboratory. When representatives from Philips Corp. were at the airport to meet him when his flight arrived he abruptly terminated his visit and took the next flight home.
6. Dr. George W. Crile had previously described closed chest cardiac compression, and both AC and DC internal defibrillation in dogs as well as humans in his book "Anemia and Resuscitation." He was able to resuscitate 3 of 10 patients who had apparently died of "pulseless collapse" in the operating room.[6] He was unable to convince the National Electric Light Association that defibrillation would be practical for use in substations. His experience was ignored or forgotten by his successors.[7]
7. This was also where younger staff and fellows would review each day's angiographic cases. Many visitors also sat along side and learned coronary anatomy including Henry Zimmerman of St. Vincent Hospital, and later, Rene Favaloro

8. Sones' secretary for many years was Elaine Clayton. At one point she became exasperated with him and resigned—a gala farewell was held in her honor. She later returned to work for him. Shortly before we moved into the new building in 1974 she became secretary to the Board of Governors, working for Wasmuth, and later Kiser. Beverly Cohn replaced Elaine as Sones' secretary for the remainder of his time at the Clinic.

9. Sheldon was attracted to the Clinic because of its preeminence in the field of hypertension, with Drs. Page, Harriet Dustan, and Eugene Poutasse. Of course the pay helped; the USPHS fellowship paid $3600 per year plus an allowance for dependants. Elsewhere, cardiology residencies paid anywhere from $25 to $250 per month, (plus meals, and lodging—if single). Married in 1958 to Margaret Demichelis, and with one son and another child on the way, they moved to a garden apartment in Euclid. By the luck of the draw his first rotation at the Clinic was in Sones' Department. Near the end of his fellowship in 1962 he was offered a junior staff position at $10,000/yr in Hypertension Research, and a Clinical Associate position at $7500/yr in Sones' Department. He chose the latter because coronary arteriography was gaining interest nationally and promised to revolutionize the treatment of coronary artery disease: myocardial revascularization surgery was beginning with coronary endarterectomies and internal mammary implants.

10. Designed by Pieter Kok of the Philips Corporation.

11. Unfortunately using this injector he lost the tactile sensation provided by a manual syringe injection, and on more than one occasion he aspirated air into the injector and injected it into a coronary artery. Fortunately no fatalities occurred. It had been learned that a few small air bubbles injected into a coronary artery rarely caused a problem except infrequently when transient bradycardia occurred. However larger injections of air caused asystole; patients were transferred to the operating room while undergoing closed chest massage. After a few such occurrences Effler and colleagues learned that opening the chest for cardiac compression and/or defibrillation was rarely necessary—with continued closed-chest external cardiac counterpulsation spontaneous cardiac activity returned after several minutes.

12. I recall one middle age woman who experienced angina after radiation therapy for breast cancer. Sones' coronary arteriography revealed very severe stenoses at the ostia of both the right and left main coronary

arteries. Sones advised immediate surgery—bilateral coronary endarterectomies—but the patient's husband was hesitant. After impassioned pleading and dire predictions of the prognosis, Sones got him to agree. Effler performed the operation which regrettably she did not survive. We had not yet appreciated the hazard of direct operations on the left coronary artery.

13. Interestingly, in April 1956, Dr. A.W. Humphries, an orthopedic surgeon at the Clinic who soon became one of the nation's first vascular surgeons, sent the following memo to the Board of Governors:

> PURPOSE: To develop an effective method of increasing blood flow to the myocardia.
>
> BACKGROUND: Intermittently prior to 1940 and with sporadic flurries since 1940 there has been work done even at clinical level to increase and to supplement blood supply to the heart. The Roberts 1 and Roberts 2 and Beck 1 procedures have been devised along this premise.
>
> Since approximately 1950, the surgical technique involving the handling of blood vessels has been enormously developed and there is an ever increasing understanding of what can and cannot be done mechanically to blood flow.
>
> The development of techniques and machinery for the handling of developmental defects of cardiac anatomy and the modification of changes in valves secondary to disease have increased the tools and the techniques available for work on the heart. The results of developing a method of increasing blood flow to the myocardia would be the opening of a new attack on the most prevalent pathologic change in the world today. The need for such a procedure is obvious. It is my opinion that medicine is on the verge of initiating this field.
>
> BREAKDOWN: This problem resolves itself into three basic components: 1) the development of diagnostic media which I presume means some form of angiography. This could manifest itself in the form of x-ray film, movie film or fluoroscopy using an iodine-bearing medium or it might be manifested by the use

of some radioactive medicine. A closed method of obtaining diagnostic criteria is, of course, to be desired. 2) the development of a technique devised to—a) replace existing coronary vessels, b) transplant new vessels or c) cause the patient to grow new vessels. The necessary equipment for the handling of vessels and the preparation and preservation and some knowledge of the technique of the use and handling is already in existence here. 3) a methodology for being able to work on the heart itself is necessary. The technique of thoracotomy, hibernation and refrigeration are all present here in this institution and if necessary, the cross-circulation equipment is in existence.

DISCUSSION: It would seem to me that the development of a method of increasing blood flow to the myocardia would be one of the most significant things the Cleveland Clinic Foundation could do at this time. I am personally convinced that this would be the next big step in surgery and it would seem to me that being a leader in this field would be of great advantage to the Clinic from a financial as well as a profitable point of view. The basic tools which would be necessary for a project such as this are probably all in existence in one form or another and the tools which would conceivably be needed are already in existence here. I should think chat with some concentrating work upon the problem that in the not too distant future certain early steps toward the development of this could be worked out in this institution.

It is suggested that this problem be considered by the Clinic to determine whether the profits to be gained from such a venture would be worth whatever amount of money had to be put into it and the time of the individual or individuals who would be involved in attempting to work this out.

The Board of Governors had been in existence barely four months when its Chairman, Dr. Fay LeFevre, answered Humphries as follows:

The Board of Governors reviewed your memorandum regarding future cardiac research in surgery. I have been informed that the project you had in mind has already been outlined and will receive consideration in the very near future. If you have any questions concerning this, I shall be glad to discuss them with you at any time.

Humphries had been tapped by Dr. George Crile Jr. and Dr. Robert Dinsmore to develop vascular surgery at the Clinic in about 1955. The Department of Vascular Surgery was established in 1957. This proposal was made just two months after Effler performed the first open heart procedure with elective cardiac arrest. Humphries' proposal died quickly. He was not trained as a thoracic surgeon, and both Sones and Effler disliked him. Ernstene was also on the Board of Governors at the time, and saw this as an attempt for him to expand into cardiac surgery.

14. This was before the era of myocardial revascularization surgery. Mainetti was impressed with Sones' work in coronary arteriography and Effler's expertise in cardiac surgery and advised Favaloro that the Clinic would be the best place to learn cardiac surgery.

15. Shirey reports that shortly before this meeting he and Sones had been investigating several contrast agents, some of which seemed arrhythmogenic. Despite Shirey's admonition to suspend this investigation during the meeting, as many physicians attending the meeting visited the laboratory, Sones persisted, and in three patients ventricular fibrillation occurred, all successfully defibrillated. An unidentified visitor remarked "They tell us the procedure is safe but they aren't telling us the truth."

16. A few years earlier I had written a paper summarizing the variety of coronary artery anomalies that had been encountered, with representative illustrations. As most of these studies had been performed before I arrived I felt it was important to have Sones' review and approval. The manuscript sat on his desk unreviewed for weeks. After repeated inquiries, he finally told me to go ahead and submit it for publication and that it was OK to use his name as an author. Absent his review the paper was never submitted.

17. Most of these men, as well as many other internationally renowned cardiologists visited Sones at the Clinic, a rare opportunity for the staff and fellows.

18. On another occasion in 1969 after Wasmuth had become Chairman of the Board of Governors, he held staff meetings in the evening,

after a cocktail reception to stimulate interest and attendance in these meetings. At one of them, in April 1969, Sones had imbibed generously at the cocktail reception, and during the subsequent meeting became vocal and critical during a presentation by H. Richard Taylor, Director of Public Affairs, castigating him severely and calling him a cheap "beer salesman." All were shocked and embarrassed and the meeting was adjourned. The next day Sones sent a personally signed letter of apology to each member of the Professional Staff. Thereafter Staff Meetings were held in the afternoon, sans alcoholic beverages

19. A few years earlier Groves anastomosed the right subclavian artery of a Labrador Retriever dog to its anterior descending artery. The dog survived and became a family pet, "Nellie," for several years. Earlier vein to coronary artery bypass grafts in humans that went unreported were performed by Sabiston (1962)[23], Garrett (1964)[24] and Kahn (1966)[25].

20. Norman Shumway of Stanford University did the second transplant in 1968.

21. The former business manager was reassigned to head a Clinic subsidiary and a short time later he died by his own hand at the Bolton Square Hotel.

22. It is probable that Wasmuth also wanted to assume responsibility for all staff salaries, but the Trustees would not agree to this since it would jeopardize the Clinic's not-for-profit status. At least "on paper" they approved all salaries.

23. Heretofore the Chairman of the Research Division was appointed by the Trustees, and reported only to the Trustees. His salary was determined by the Trustees, and it was rumored that he had a unique retirement plan with a fixed salary for life. He was the only professional employee of the Clinic to have this status. This changed after Wasmuth became Chairman, and he was now treated as any other Division Chairman.

24. "Cost-plus" reimbursement was still provided by Medicare and Blue Cross.

25. Turnbull, a popular surgeon and deeply committed to the Clinic, was not pleased with the new policy and resigned and moved to California to begin a new practice.

26. Mac Evarts, Dick Farmer, Dub Gifford, Bruce Stewart, Bill Kiser, Sheldon and others participated in these discussions. See also reference to a suggested cardiovascular division in Note 15, The Sheldon Years.

27. Internal mammary to anterior descending anastomoses had first been promulgated by George Greene of New York (1968). Favaloro had used the internal mammary artery on two occasions which were both unsuccessful. Loop resurrected it in January, 1971.

28. In earlier years Sones and Proudfit had contemplated the need for a means of codifying clinical and angiographic data for correlative purposes. Sones had learned in Washington that a grant might be found for such a project. Dr. Peter Kwiterovich, a lipidologist from Johns Hopkins Medical School was sent to Cleveland to assess the feasibility. Impressed with the potential for a database, and with Sones' detailed catheterization reports he suggested (1) more detailed information regarding serum lipids be included and (2) that a full time director be sought and (3) that the project be under the auspices of the NIH. Sones saw this as an attempt to control the data and rejected it.

29. The CVIR database was later transferred to the Clinic's VAX computer, and still later to its IBM mainframe computer. Since its inception the CVIR has been funded directly from Clinic revenues, as is the Cancer Registry.

Eugene Blackstone, M.D. became Director of the CVIR in October, 1997. With the development of several databases in Cardiology and Cardiac Surgery, the CVIR maintains its own dedicated database of patient information, and draws on other integrated registries for procedural data: cardiac catheterization, interventional, echocardiography, heart failure, and others. The CVIR continues to acquire followup information on several thousand coronary bypass, valve surgery, thoracic aneurysm and cardiac transplant patients each year. It regularly provides procedural and outcome data to other national registries including the STS (Society for Thoracic Surgery) registry. The CVIR database currently includes over 194,000 patients, 200,000 cardiac catheterizations and 120,000 surgical procedures.

30. See also Chapter 3.

31. Proudfit recalls:

> Wasmuth suggested that I supervise the drawing of plans for the first floor of the new cardiology building and that Sones should be responsible for the second floor. My job was relatively simple—almost entirely drawing the dimensions of

the offices and examining rooms and the electrocardiographic section. Sones had a much more complex task, because of the new catheterization laboratories. Mason and I agreed that provisions should be made for adding additional floors to the building to allow for expansion. I determined that the minimum size of the examining rooms were 120 square feet. After construction we went around to find that the architects had shrunk the size of the examining rooms to 80 square feet. This was uncomfortably small and allowed easy access to the patient from only one side during physical examination, either the right or left. Most cardiologists prefer to stand to the right of the patient but some, notably Wayne Siegel, liked the left side. I had no preference, but the rooms were so small that it was difficult to get around. Mason was furious and demanded that the builders modify the rooms on the second floor. He wanted to use one room for interviewing the patient or giving reports, and an adjacent room for physical examination. Of course, this design negated the original purpose—providing the maximum number of rooms. So on the first floor we had uncomfortably small examining rooms and on the second floor the number of rooms was inadequate. Mason and I should have inspected the blueprints more carefully and insisted on the original dimensions, but we trusted the architects. At least we had the promise that additional floors could be added when needed. Unfortunately, when this occasion arose, we were told that the foundation would not support additional floors!

32. A new Research Building was completed in 1973. The Park Plaza Inn on E 96h St. was completed in 1974
33. It was in the early 1970s that Wasmuth named Effler head of a "Resource Utilization Committee." Effler seized the charge with a passion and looked into needless expenditures throughout all Departments. When he eliminated the coffee maker from the surgeons' lounge he met a rebellion and it was not long before the effort quietly disappeared.
34. As I recall it, Proudfit was on the B/G when the Board changed the policy and required that Department Heads step down at age 60. This was because Effler was unpopular. Rupert Turnbull, Chairman of Colorectal Surgery, was the first to be affected by this policy, and

he soon left the Clinic for California. Proudfit was next, and stepped down at age 60 in 1974. Effler would be next, but that left only Sones as the only remaining member of the triumvirate to remain as a Department Head—an unsatisfactory situation for Effler, as well as several members of Proudfit's Department whom Sones had berated. The Board appointed search committees for cardiology and thoracic and cardiovascular surgery. (There was only one search committee for Cardiology—for Proudfit's successor—chaired by Dub Gifford.) Ralph Straffon chaired the cardiac surgery search committee. Now that the two departments of cardiology had been brought together geographically they would be able to function better together and it no longer seemed appropriate to have two separate cardiology training programs—(integration of the two training programs was already beginning to happen, the result of discussions at the Tri-Departmental meetings). Some of the members of the two Departments of cardiology suggested combining them into a single entity. Upon recommendation of the Search Committee, the Board determined that the two Departments would be amalgamated; Proudfit, Sones and Effler became interim Chairmen.

Sones was suspicious that Sheldon had actively sought his position, which is incorrect; (I had always admired Sones and considered him a good friend, but recognized the Sones-Effler conflict had reached an impasse and also that Sones could not be a good leader for all the members of Proudfit's Department. Wayne Siegel was the one who first approached me regarding the chairmanship and I was noncommittal). Sones made an impassioned appearance before the Board indicating that he did not wish to step down. Shirey also appeared before the Board in favor of maintaining the status quo, retaining Sones as head of his department, and finding a successor for Proudfit. The cardiology search committee made its report a few weeks earlier than the cardiac surgery search committee. Wasmuth and Gifford announced the report and Board's decision of the cardiology search committee to all the members of the two departments in the conference room next to Wasmuth's office. I sat next to Shirey at this meeting. Although he had been a reluctant candidate for the chairmanship—only if amalgamation was inevitable—and he was disappointed to see this happen. Our close friendship continues to this day.

35. I was present when Effler responded to Wasmuth's request to meet with him late one afternoon in the B/G office. Impeccably dressed as usual, he entered regally, addressing Wasmuth rather characteristically as "Your corpulence." Wasmuth pleaded with Effler to remain at the Clinic, in any capacity he wished. He mentioned Directorship of the International Center. Effler responded that he planned to continue surgery into his 80s or 90s, as his father had, and that he was committed to leaving.

36. On creating a window between the pericardial and pleural spaces for the management of pericardial effusion.

37. I highly recommend Favaloro's monograph *The Challenging Dream of Heart Surgery. From the Pampus to Cleveland*, 1992, (Reference 20, Chapter 1) It provides unique insights into not only his personality, and his life through the Cleveland Clinic years, but also his friendships with Effler, Sones and Proudfit.

38. Sones previously underwent a left carotid endarterectomy. He had experienced transient dysarthria, and made the diagnosis himself, confirming it when he auscultated his neck and noted a carotid bruit. The operation was performed by Dr. Edwin Beven of the Department of Vascular Surgery.

39. A new primary is a more accurate description. The previous cancerous nodule was deemed to have been cured by complete excision.

40. When Proudfit inquired of Sones if he had received Tizard's letters he had no knowledge of them. Jokingly, Proudfit said that he must remember Galen, knowing that Mason had no interest in medical history. Sones smiled and said, "Galen, Galen, I remember him. I was number 61 in my graduating class in medical school and Galen was number 62."

References for The Proudfit-Sones Years

1. Zimmerman HA. Scott RW. Becker NO: Catheterization of the left side of the heart in man. Circulation. 1950;1(3):357-9.

2. Bailey, CP: The surgical treatment of mitral stenosis (mitral commissurotomy). Dis Chest. 1949;15:377.

3. Harken, DE, Ellis, LB, Ware, PF and Norman, LR: The surgical treatment of mitral stenosis. I, Valvuloplasty. New Engl J Med. 1948;239:801.

4. Sones FM Jr, Shirey EK, Proudfit WL, and Westcott, RN: Cine-coronary arteriography. (abst) Circulation. 1959;20:773.

5. Kouwenhoven, WB, Jude JR and Knickerbocker GG: Closed-chest cardiac massage. JAMA. 1960;173:1064.

6. Wiggers, HW. *Anemia and Resuscitation*. New York and London: D. Appleton & Co; 1914.

7. Proudfit WL. Personal communication, 2005.

8. Sones FM Jr and Shirey EK: Cine Coronary Arteriography. Mod Concept Cardiovasc. Dis. 1962;31:735-738.

9. Sheldon WC: Unpublished conversations with William L. Proudfit. 2005.

10. Nouse DC: Letter to the author, July 15, 1994.

11. Effler DB, Groves LK, Sones FM Jr, Shirey EK: Increased myocardial perfusion by internal mammary artery implant: Vineberg's operation. Ann Surg. 1963;Oct;158:526-36.

12. Favaloro RG, Effler DB, Groves LK, Fergusson DJ, Lozada JS: Double internal mammary artery-myocardial implantation. Clinical evaluation of results in 150 patients. Circulation. 1968;Apr;37(4):549-55.

13. Fergusson DJ, Shirey EK, Sheldon, WC, et al: Left internal mammary implant—post-operative assessment. Circulation. 1969;37 & 38(Supp 1):61.

14. Fergusson DJ, Shirey EK, Sheldon WC, Effler DB and Sones FM Jr: Left internal mammary artery implant—postoperative assessment. Circulation. l968;37-38, II-24.

15. Shirey EK, Sones FM Jr: Retrograde transaortic and mitral valve catheterization. Physiologic and morphologic evaluation of aortic and mitral valve lesions. Am J Cardiol. 1966; Nov;18(5):745-53.

16. Likoff W, Segal BL, Kasparian H: Paradox of normal selective coronary arteriograms in patients considered to have unmistakable coronary heart disease. N Engl J Med. 1967;May 11;276(19):1063-6.

17. Shirey EK, Hawk WA, Mukerji D, Effler DB: Percutaneous myocardial biopsy of the left ventricle. Experience in 198 patients. Circulation. 1972; Jul;46(1):112-22.

18. Shirey EK, Proudfit WL, Hawk, WA: Primary myocardial disease. Correlation with clinical findings, angiographic and biopsy diagnosis. Follow-up of 139 patients. Am Heart J. 1980;99(2):198-207.

19. Proudfit WL, Shirey EK, Sones FM Jr: Selective cine coronary arteriography. Correlation with clinical findings in 1,000 patients. Circulation. 1966; Jun;33(6):901-910.

20. Proudfit WL, Shirey EK, Sones FM Jr: Distribution of arterial lesions demonstrated by selective cinecoronary arteriography. Circulation. 1967: Jul;36(1):54-62.

21. Proudfit WL, Shirey EK, Sheldon WC, Sones FM Jr: Certain clinical characteristics correlated with extent of obstructive lesions demonstrated by selective cine-coronary arteriography. Circulation. 1968:Nov;38(5):947-54.

22. Flores MC, Proudfit WL, Shirey EK: Inferior myocardial infarction. Correlation of selective cine coronary arteriographic and ventriculographic findings with form of QRS complex in lead AVF. Cleve Clin Q. 1973; Spring;40(1):15-20.

23. Sabiston DC Jr: The coronary circulation. Johns Hopkins Med J. 1974; 134:314-329.

24. Garrett HE, Dennis EW and DeBakey ME: Aortocoronary bypass with saphenous vein graft. JAMA. 1973;223:792-794.

25. Kahn D: Discussion of paper: The simple approach to direct coronary artery surgery. The Cleveland Clinic experience. Effler DB, Favaloro RG, Groves LK, Loop FD. J Thorac Cardiovasc Surg. 1971; 62:509.

26. Favaloro RG: Saphenous vein autograft replacement of severe segmental coronary artery occlusion: operative technique. Ann Thorac Surg. 1968;Apr;5(4):334-9.

27. Favaloro RG, Effler DB, Cheanvechai CH, Quint RA Sones FM Jr: Acute coronary insufficiency (impending myocardial infarction and myocardial infarction). Surgical treatment by the saphenous vein technique. Am J Cardiol. 1971;28:598-607.

28. Green GE, Stertzer, SH, Reppert EH: Coronary arterial bypass grafts. Ann Thorac Surg. 1968;5:443.

29. Judkins, MP: Selective cine coronary arteriography. Part I. A percutaneous femoral technic. Radiol. 1967,89:815-824.

30. Wasmuth CE: Personal communication, 1988.

31. Bruschke AV, Proudfit WL, Sones FM Jr: Clinical course of patients with normal, and slightly or moderately abnormal coronary arteriograms. A follow-up study on 500 patients. Circulation. 1973; May;47(5):936-45.

32. Bruschke AVG, Proudfit WL, Sones FM: Progress study of 590 consecutive non-surgical cases of coronary disease followed 5-9 years. I. Arteriographic correlations. Circulation. 1973;47:1147.

33. Bruschke AVG, Proudfit WL, Sones FMS Jr: Progress study of 590 consecutive nonsurgical cases of coronary disease followed 5-9 years. II. Ventriculographic and other correlations Circulation. 1973 Jun;47(6):1154-63.

34. Proudfit WL, Bruschke AV, Sones FM Jr: Natural history of obstructive coronary artery disease. Supplement to a 10-year study. Cleve Clin Q. 1978;Winter;45(4):293-8.

35. Proudfit WL, Bruschke AV, Sones FM Jr: Natural history of obstructive coronary artery disease: ten-year study of 601 nonsurgical cases. Prog Cardiovasc Dis. 1978;Jul-Aug;21(1):53-78.

36. Proudfit WL, Bruschke VG, Sones FM Jr: Clinical course of patients with normal or slightly or moderately abnormal coronary arteriograms: 10-year follow-up of 521 patients. Circulation. 1980; Oct;62(4):712-7.

37. Loop FD, Effler DB, Spampinato N, Groves LK, Cheanvechai C: Myocardial revascularization by internal mammary artery grafts. A technique without optical assistance. J Thorac Cardiovasc Surg. 1972;Apr;63(4):674-80.

38. Loop FD, Spampinato N, Siegel, W and Effler DB: Internal mammary artery grafts without optical assistance. Clinical and Angiographic analysis of 175 consecutive cases. Circulation. 1973; 47 & 48 (Supp III): 162-167.

39. Moberg CH, Webster JS, Sones FM Jr.: Natural history of severe proximal coronary disease as defined by angiography (abstr). Presented at 21st Scientific Session, American College of Cardiology (Chicago, March 3, 1972). Amer J Cardiol. 1972;29:282.

40. Webster JS, Moberg C, Rincon G: Natural history of severe proximal coronary artery disease as documented by coronary cineangiography. Am J. Cardiol. 1974;33:195.

41. SheldonWC, Sones FM Jr, Shirey EK, Fergusson DJG, Favaloro RG and Effler DB: Reconstructive coronary artery surgery: postoperative assessment. Circulation. 1969; 39 & 40(Suppl. I):61.

42. Sheldon WC, Rincon, G, Effler DB, Proudfit WL, and Sones FM Jr.: Vein graft surgery for coronary artery disease. Survival and angiographic results in 1,000 patients. Circulation. 1973; Suppl III, 47 & 48; III:184.

43. Sheldon WC, Rincon G, Pichard AD, Razavi M, Cheanvechai C, and Loop FD: Surgical treatment of coronary artery disease: Pure graft operations, with a study of 741 patients followed 3-7 yr. Progr in Cardiov Dis. 1975;18:237.

44. Siegel, W. Personal communication, June 25, 2006.

45. Heupler FA Jr, Proudfit WL, Siegel, et al: The ergonovine maleate test for the diagnosis of coronary artery spasm (Abst). Circulation. 1975;52 (Supp. II):11.
46. Proudfit WL: The Fleece Medical Society. Br Heart J. 1981;46:589,
47. Proudfit WL: John Hunter: on heart disease. Br Heart J. 1986;Aug; 56(2):109-14.
48. Proudfit WL: John Fothergill and angina pectoris. Br Heart J. 1991; Oct;66(4):322-4.

THE SHELDON YEARS
1975-1991

Sheldon inherited two outstanding, highly specialized and complex departments that had evolved over the previous fifteen years under the leadership of Proudfit and Sones. At the time of the amalgamation there were 18 staff physicians: eight in Clinical Cardiology and ten in the Department of Cardiovascular Disease and the Cardiac Catheterization Laboratory; Neil Hart and Ernesto Salcedo had joined the staff in Clinical Cardiology earlier in 1975, as did John Kramer, Khosrow Dorosti and Irving Franco in the Cardiac Laboratory. There were eleven special fellows in Clinical Cardiology and 31 in the cath lab—for a total of 42, the largest cardiology program in the country. New technology was emerging. Sheldon, known more for his organizational ability than for his charisma, was charged with the task of integrating these departments into a workable entity that preserved their strengths and improved their organization, communication, and functionality.

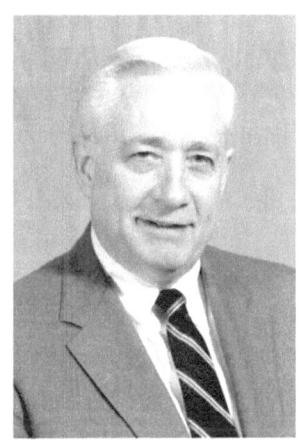

William C. Sheldon

Hart, a graduate of Saint Louis University School of Medicine and the Clinic's Internal Medicine Program, did his cardiology training in Atlanta, and then returned to join Proudfit's Department. He excelled as a teacher and was highly regarded by the fellows. He became a vice-chairman of the Education Committee, program director for the non-invasive training program, and coordinator of the internal medicine rotator teaching service. He left for private practice in Pittsburgh in 1982 where he expanded his practice into invasive and interventional cardiology.

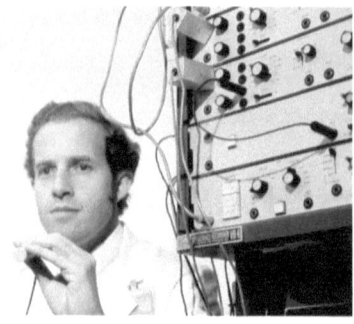

Ernesto E. Salcedo

Ernesto Salcedo, a Peruvian by birth, was a graduate of the Internal Medicine program at the University of Connecticut, and a cardiology fellowship at Cleveland Metropolitan General Hospital. He came to the Clinic as a Clinical Associate and Advanced Research Fellow of the Cleveland Chapter of the American Heart Association in 1974. He worked with Siegel in the Cardiac Function Laboratory assessing left ventricular function with echocardiography, later succeeding him as Head of the Cardiac Function Laboratory after Siegel left in 1977. He built that laboratory into a large nationally renowned entity. It became the center of the Clinic's noninvasive cardiac imaging that would later collaborate with Radiology's Department of Nuclear Medicine in imaging modalities that included nuclear, Cardiac CT, and MRI. Salcedo published two textbooks on cardiac echocardiography; he later chaired the Cardiology Research Committee.

Kramer was a graduate of the University of Virginia Medical School, and the Clinic's training programs in Internal Medicine and Cardiovascular Disease. He later married a cath lab nurse. He became interested in laser applications in the catheterization laboratory and developed the Laser Research Laboratory, working closely with the Massachusetts Institute of Technology. He published extensively and traveled widely. He became an early critic of coronary angioplasty as it later evolved at the Clinic.

Dorosti was a native of Iran, and a graduate of the Clinic's fellowship in Cardiovascular Disease. He became a steady, reliable worker with excellent cath lab skills and a good teacher. He was among the first to learn angioplasty technics as they evolved. Franco was a native of the Dominican Republic and a graduate of the Clinic's fellowship in Cardiovascular Disease who was also a dedicated tireless worker. He too would become one of the early interventional cardiologists.

The new South Clinic, designed in collaboration with Sones and Proudfit, provided a modern new facility around which the new Department would be structured [1]: the catheterizing cardiologists (soon to be called "invasive cardiologists") were located on the second floor (Desk F25) [2], next to the catheterization laboratories on the second floor of the adjacent hospital building (Desk F26) where Lucille Vanderwyst continued as head Nurse [3]; Clinical Cardiology ("noninvasive cardiologists") was on the first floor (Desk F15), adjacent to the ECG Laboratory (Claudette Matero, Supervisor), and the new Cardiac Function Laboratory ("noninvasive" echocardiography and ECG-stress testing laboratories—Jean McIntosh, Supervisor) (Desk F16); this was a part of the Cardiology Outpatient Testing Center that also included blood drawing facilities for laboratory Medicine, and a chest x-ray facility for the Division of Radiology—Radiology was located immediately below, in the basement of the new building.

A satellite ECG laboratory was retained at Desk 81, (Nora Slater, Supervisor), to serve the Main Clinic building. A new ECG satellite was established in the West Clinic (old Clinic Inn) to serve the Primary Care and Executive Health Departments. The new ECG Lab on the first floor (Desk 16) served hospital patients as well as Cardiology outpatients in the South Clinic building.

The offices for Cardiac Surgery were also at F-25, and the cardiac operating rooms were in a remodeled area on the second floor of the hospital, not far from the cardiac intensive care and coronary intensive care units on the second floor of the new hospital building. In effect, the cath labs were close to the coronary intensive care unit as well as the operating rooms. The invasive cardiologists were at F25 next to the cath labs (except Sones wanted his office to be within the Cath Lab area), the clinical cardiologists were at F15 next to the ECG, echo and stress labs and not far from the CICU. It was an ideal arrangement for all.

A New Structure for a New Department

The basic functioning units of cardiology were preserved in the form of sections, with their easily identifiable leaders.

> **Section of Clinical Cardiology**—Desk 15: Royston Lewis
> **Section of Cardiac Catheterization**—Desk 25 and Desk 26:
> Earl Shirey

Section of the Cardiac Function Laboratory: Wayne Siegel—
(Salcedo became Head after Siegel moved to Florida in
May 1977)
Section of Electrocardiography: Royston Lewis

The Section of Pacemakers and Electrophysiology was formalized in 1976 with Lon Castle as its Director. Permanent pacemakers, His-bundle studies and M-mode cardiac ultrasound studies were fledgling technologies in 1975 but monumental advances would emerge within the next decade. Room five of the new cath lab complex became the Pacemaker Laboratory and an outpatient Pacemaker Center that included a Pacemaker Registry was set up in an office at Desk 15.

Before the move into the new facilities took place, Effler had suggested that Mr. John Florio, a coordinator in the surgical intensive care unit, might be helpful to Sones as an administrative assistant. Sones hired him at B-10 and he began to work on the rather chaotic appointment making system and secretarial typing pool. In the new facility he became Departmental Administrator for F-25 and the Cardiac Catheterization Laboratories and Ms. Marjorie Horn became Administrator of the newly created Cardiology Appointment Desk (Desk F12, later F-14), and ultimately became responsible also for Desks F-15 and F-16.

Cardiology Department Meetings were held each month, and the Tri-Departmental forums continued. A Daily Information Sheet was distributed to all Staff and supervisors detailing each day's conference schedule, on-call assignments, surgical and catheterization schedules, and hospital census information. For the first time Cardiology Annual Reports were produced and distributed to all Cardiology staff with complete disclosure of productivity and financial data, cath lab complications, and a summary of educational and research activities, and publications. [4]

As the members of the new Department pursued their various interests and clinical practices they began to plan for an even stronger Department. Sheldon established a committee structure to aid in the organization and governance of the Department. This was the new era of participatory management. [5]

With the supportive relationships that had been built between the departments of Cardiology, Thoracic and Cardiovascular Surgery and

Cardiothoracic Anesthesiology, the geographic proximity of these departments with their clinic and hospital components in the new buildings, and the operational infrastructure in Cardiology—appointment making, secretarial support and fiscal management—all designed to provide efficient patient care, the *integrated cardiovascular practice unit* was in place.[1] It proved to be a highly successful model that was key to the growth of the cardiovascular program in the years ahead.

A **Cardiology Education Committee** was created to integrate the separate cardiology training programs into a combined program. Mehdi Razavi was Chairman of this Committee and Neil Hart and Fred Heupler served as Co-Program Directors for the Noninvasive and Invasive training programs respectively. James Hodgman, who continued to organize the Saturday morning Cardiology Grand Rounds, Lewis, and Shirey were also members of the Education Committee. The Education Committee set about defining suitable rotations that would meet the needs of the fellows interested in catheterization, as well as those interested in clinical cardiology. Many new diagnostic and therapeutic modalities—beyond electrocardiography, ECG-stress testing and cardiac catheterization—were beginning to emerge that had to be accommodated in the fellowship training programs. Under the guidance of the Education Committee, Cardiology continued to sponsor regular postgraduate courses, and many well-known speakers and visiting professors attended conferences and postgraduate courses.

As cardiology rotations for internal medicine fellows had been discontinued years before, these fellows had no exposure to cardiology; but in 1975 these rotations were resumed. Although the help of internal medicine rotators in the hospital and with night and weekend coverage was enthusiastically welcomed, the Education Committee had to structure a meaningful educational program for them. There was no strategy for including congenital heart disease in the training program. A **Congenital Heart Disease Clinic** was developed by Drs. Shirey, Razavi, Lardani and Hart with the hope that clustering congenital heart disease patients in a weekly clinic would offer a better teaching experience for our fellows.

The **Coronary Intensive Care Committee** consisted of Jim Hodgman, Chairman, Lon Castle and Dan Phillips. Although our coronary intensive care was modest in comparison to those in other hospitals,—our referral practice brought relatively few patients with acute myocardial infarction—coronary intensive care units were becoming more sophisticated and were beginning to offer hemodynamic monitoring and Swan-Ganz pulmonary artery catheterizations. Academia had their myocardial infarction research units (MIRU's).

A **Cardiology Research Committee** was created with Proudfit as its Chairman, and included Juan Lim, Loop and Sheldon. This Committee also acted as the advisory committee to the Cardiovascular Information Registry (Emily Wagstaff continued as its work leader.) Loop also continued his interest in the CVIR.

Wayne Siegel explored M-mode ultrasound studies of the heart with unidimensional transducers. A single laboratory for echocardiography had been included in the first floor at F-16, adjacent to the ECG Department. Soon two more echocardiography laboratories were added. A gamma camera was donated to the Department by Mr. Ray Firestone of the Firestone Tire and Rubber Co. and Gustavo Rincon began to work with Dr. Bill McIntyre of the Division of Radiology in nuclear cardiac imaging using thallium-201. These were the roots of what would soon become substantial noninvasive imaging modalities in Cardiology.

An intraäortic balloon pump had recently been acquired by the Department of Thoracic and Cardiovascular Surgery but was seldom used. Daniel Philips learned about the equipment and began to use it for patients who "crashed" in the intensive care unit. It was not long before Cardiac Surgery took over this responsibility.

Loop's first additions to the Department of Thoracic and Cardiovascular Surgery were Delos Cosgrove (1975) and Bruce Lytle (1978). Both came from training in cardiac surgery at Massachusetts General Hospital and immediately proved to be skilled and innovative surgeons. Cosgrove spent several weeks

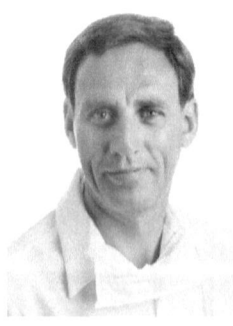
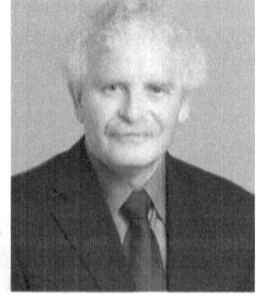

Delos M. "Toby" Cosgrove   Bruce W. Lytle

in the early 1980s with Prof Alain Carpentier in Paris France learning about mitral valve repair. Cautiously he began to perform mitral valvuloplasties at the Clinic, and it was not long before he became the nation's leading advocate of valve repair surgery.[2,3]

The Cleveland Clinic International Center for Specialty Studies

Sheldon continued as a member of the Board of Governors from 1975-1980. During this time he chaired several search committees and review committees. The Cleveland Clinic had always enjoyed somewhat of an international reputation, and several physicians had often been invited to lecture at foreign meetings and medical centers, going back to the days of George Crile Sr. Sheldon had been invited to be keynote speaker at the annual meeting of the Philippine Heart Association, and observed the high regard with which the Clinic was held by local cardiologists. Upon returning to Cleveland he proposed in June 1975 that a formal international program be established, with the objective of promoting physician exchanges with established foreign centers for educational purposes. The Board adopted the proposal, but it was not until Saudi Arabian King Khaled presented a grant of $500,000 to the Clinic, that it became economically feasible. Wasmuth proposed that the grant be directed to this international exchange program, and suggested its name: "The Cleveland Clinic International Center for Specialty Studies."[6] An advisory committee was appointed, and guidelines were developed, and Sheldon was named Chairman in December 1975, a post he held until 1987 when he transferred the leadership to Mehdi Razavi. This was the first formal program in any U.S. medical center to provide opportunities for foreign physicians to visit this country to learn and observe. In return, increasing numbers of Clinic Staff members were invited to participate in foreign meetings and lectureships with the support of the International Center. By 1987 more than 350 physicians and paramedical personnel from more than 40 countries had visited the Clinic. Fifty Clinic Staff members had visited foreign centers on teaching assignments and visiting professorships, and the Clinic had co-sponsored 27 international symposia. Nineteen of our Fellows had received International Traveling Fellowship Awards. In addition the International Center became a vehicle to facilitate referral of patients from foreign centers to the Clinic, and provided assistance with local travel, appointments, interpreters, etc.—more than 2600 patients from 80 countries in 1987. Formal or informal affiliations had been developed with the Philippine Heart Center for Asia, the Intermed Clinic, an outpatient cardiology clinic in Istanbul, Turkey, Ain Shams University in Cairo, Egypt and the King Faisal Specialist Hospital in Rabat, Saudi Arabia and the Clinic now has continuing relationships also with centers in United Arab Emirates, Singapore, Canada, and Vienna. [7]

In 1976, despite achieving a record number of cardiac catheterizations (over 6,000 annually), the waiting list for caths also reached an all time high, 784, as did the waiting list for cardiac surgery, nearly 300. The internal mammary artery had been used as a bypass graft to the anterior descending artery since 1971, and within two years its superior graft patency was evident. Surgical referrals grew, and a third of surgical patients were "mail order patients"—those who were studied elsewhere and referred directly to the cardiac surgeons. [8] Hospital occupancy was 93 percent, and cardiology beds were insufficient to accommodate our patients and increasing numbers went to non-cardiology floors. The five-bed Coronary Intensive Care Unit proved to be too small and many patients were admitted to the surgical ICU "Blue Room" next door, or to the Medical Intensive Care Unit. [9] All this was within two years after occupying the new hospital and clinic facilities.

In 1976 the Education Committee began to grapple with strategies to reduce the size of the training program, which had become the largest in the country, and ways of achieving a more favorable balance between foreign graduates (92 percent of fellows) vs. American graduates. It was recognized that the need for additional fellows had in part been dictated by a growing staff, and the service demands imposed upon fellows were becoming counterproductive to an optimal training experience. In addition there were threats from academia to curtail non-academic training programs. We decided not to participate in the National Cardiology Fellowship Matching Plan, but continue our independent recruitment process. A brochure was developed for potential fellowship candidates.

All former Cardiology fellows were surveyed in 1976 to obtain their views of their training experience. Sixty-five of 123 responded.

ABIM certified	89%
CVD certified	89%

Caths performed in 1975	12,000
No. holding med school appointments	19
Directors of Cath Labs	10

In September 1976 Wasmuth retired to Arizona and William S. Kiser, Executive Vice Chairman of the Board of Governors, was named Chairman. [10]

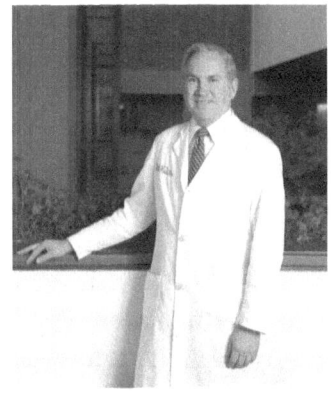

William S. Kiser

Beginning in 1977, in order to reduce the need for fellows in the cath lab so that they might have more opportunities for other rotations, selected cath lab nurses were trained to do cutdowns, incision closures and dictate portions of the catheterization report.They became known as Departmental Assistant III's (DA-III). Previously, corpsmen trained as RN's set the precedent by assisting cardiac surgeons in the operating rooms. This was the first time nurses had been used for specialized roles in patient care outside of the operating room.

In 1977 Lardani returned to Argentina and Siegel left for private practice in Florida. Ernesto Salcedo replaced Siegel as Director of the Cardiac Function Laboratory. [11] By this time portable ultrasound equipment made bedside echocardiograms possible in the hospital, and phased-array ultrasound transducers were introduced that permitted motion studies of cardiac structures, and ultimately two-dimensional echocardiography. By 1977 radionuclear-stress studies with thallium[201] and technetium[99] had become standard diagnostic tools and were no longer developmental. The gamma camera was moved to Radiology's Department of Nuclear Medicine in the basement of the South Clinic building. Treadmill ECG's were done in the Cardiac Function Laboratory at F16 after which the patient was injected with the radioactive marker and taken immediately to the Nuclear Medicine laboratory one floor below for thallium imaging. Later, Tony Cook and Ray Go took over the Nuclear Imaging laboratory. On several occasions we considered recruiting a nuclear cardiologist and launching a nuclear laboratory and training program in Cardiology, but this was opposed by Radiology. This joint Cardiology/Nuclear Radiology collaboration worked well however.

Another joint venture involved Cardiology and the Department of Orthopedic Surgery. Lon Castle had been working with Dr. John Bergfeld as team physicians for the Cleveland Browns. Bergfeld was interested in developing a fitness center for other athletes as a part of his Section of Sports Medicine. Treadmill ECG testing was to become a part of this Center, and Castle was to be co-director. After two years of discussion this was finally launched in 1981.

Pediatric Cardiology Returns

The pediatric cardiology experience for fellows in the Congenital Heart Disease Clinic, and even opportunities provided for fellows to rotate to other hospitals for pediatric cardiology fell short of our goals for the training program. We decided in 1976 to reëstablish a pediatric cardiology program and recruit a pediatric cardiologist. Carl Gill, a Mayo trained cardiac surgeon with pediatric experience, joined the Department of Thoracic and Cardiovascular Surgery in 1977. As candidates were interviewed for pediatric cardiology it became apparent that a dedicated pediatric cath lab with biplane angiographic capability would be necessary. To accommodate this, the Pacemaker/electrophysiology laboratory was transferred to Room 6.

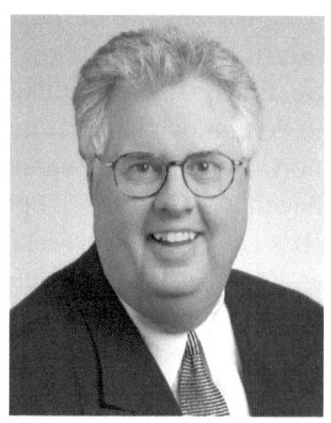

Douglas A. Moodie

Douglas Moodie, a charismatic Mayo trained pediatric cardiologist joined the Cardiology staff in 1978. With Moodie and Gill pediatric cardiology and cardiac surgery blossomed. Procedure Room 5 was dedicated to pediatric cardiology, and the new Philips Optimus 17-200 biplane angiographic equipment was installed in 1979.

The Society for Cardiac Angiography

Coronary arteriography and coronary bypass surgery were rapidly growing procedures in the United States and federal officials, health planners (Peer Review Standards organizations—PRSO's) and some cardiology leaders had become increasingly concerned of their costs to the economy and their potential for misapplication. Strategies to control these technologies were openly debated, including the establishment of restrictive indications for coronary arteriography and controlling Medicare and other third party reimbursement. In many discussions with Sones we lamented the poor performance and interpretation of coronary arteriograms in many institutions, but also the threats by health planners to promulgate restrictive indications for coronary arteriography. We also shared a concern that national cardiology and radiology organizations had failed to recognize these looming intrusions or support this growing technology. We arranged to discuss our concerns with Melvin P. Judkins, a Loma Linda radiologist who had developed a percutaneous method for coronary arteriography.[4] On November 16, 1976, we met together over dinner at the Executive House Hotel in Miami Beach, Florida during the annual meeting of the American Heart Association. Then perceived to be archrivals, it was the first time that Sones and Judkins had ever had a leisurely private conversation. They found that they had many common interests and concerns. Although nothing was resolved at that time, that conversation led to further discussions and formative meetings with leading angiographers, from both cardiology and radiology disciplines. In January 1978, in Chicago, The Society for Cardiac Angiography was launched with Sones as its first President and Sheldon as Secretary.[5,6] The SCA initiated the first large multi-institutional registry of cardiac catheterization procedures in the United States that provided a benchmark for performance. It established standards for performance, guidelines for organization of catheterization laboratories, guidelines for training programs, and for procedural indications. In a few years the Society recognized the emerging specialty of interventional cardiology after Grüntzig's introduction of percutaneous coronary angioplasty in 1977. Now known as the Society for Cardiovascular Angiography and Interventions, it now has in excess of 3000 members and is the largest international organization dedicated to quality and safety in cardiac catheterization laboratories.

In September 1977 the report of the Veterans Administration randomized study of coronary bypass surgery was published in the New England Journal of Medicine.[7] This highly publicized study concluded there was no role for bypass surgery in patients with chronic stable angina pectoris, except in the subgroup with severe disease involving the left main coronary artery.[8] Despite its flaws, it was the first randomized study of bypass surgery, and it had a profound effect on the medical community. Its impact was enhanced by a sluggish economy. Referrals dropped precipitously, and the waiting list for catheterizations fell from a high of 784 in 1976 to 300 in 1977, and the surgical waiting list dropped from 300 in 1976 to 71 in 1977. After a two-year plateau in catheterization and surgical procedures the recovery began in 1979. Subsequent reports from the VA somewhat tempered the conclusions of the initial study and identified subgroups of patients that seemed to benefit from surgery.[9] In addition other randomized studies began to appear that also showed a benefit from surgery in certain subgroups: the European Cooperative Study,[10] and in CASS (Coronary Artery Surgery Study).[11,12]

Our letter to the editor of the *New England Journal of Medicine* regarding the VA Cooperative Study was rejected and we published our rebuttals elsewhere.[13-15]

The Grüntzig Era and the Birth of Interventional Cardiology

Andreas Grüntzig, a young German cardiologist working in Zurich, had heard about Dotter's work in opening occluded leg arteries. For two years he had been working on a balloon catheter that might be used in the heart. He had been "dottering" peripheral arteries, but received no encouragement from his superiors. After visiting Richard Myler in San Francisco in May 1977 where they performed four intra-operative dilatations of stenosed coronary arteries with Grüntzig's catheter, he returned to Zurich hoping to find a suitable patient. On September 16, 1977, Grüntzig performed the first successful percutaneous dilation of a severe stenosis in the anterior descending coronary artery of a 38-year old man who had refused to undergo bypass surgery.[16] A second case a month later, with Martin Kaltenbach in Frankfurt, was unsuccessful. [12] A third, and a fourth, also with Kaltenbach,—in Zurich and Frankfurt—were successful.

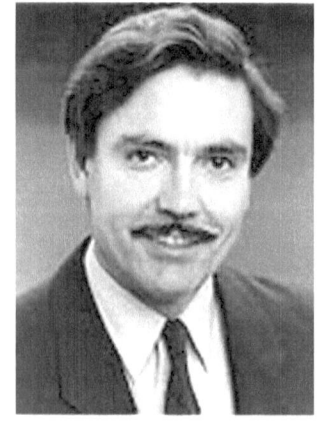

Andreas R. Grüntzig

He reported this experience at the annual scientific session of the American Heart Association in Miami, in November 1977. He showed the angiogram of the first patient. The effect was electrifying, and the large audience erupted in applause. Sones, tears streaming down both cheeks, hurried down the aisle to embrace the somewhat startled Grüntzig. (Sones had previously attempted to recanalize an occluded right coronary artery with a catheter stylus on September 16, 1964—unsuccessfully, and in the early 1970's he had devised a catheter with a rotating tip ("rotorooter") with Mr. Lowell Edwards who had created the Starr-Edwards mechanical prosthetic valve. The rotorooter catheter also proved to be unsuccessful.)

From that moment Sones and Grüntzig became close friends. Grüntzig began to hold regular teaching/demonstration seminars in Zurich that were attended by hundreds of cardiologists from around the world. Sones attended several of them, (as did Heupler and Phillips in 1980). Although there were skeptics, we resolved to explore coronary angioplasty at the Clinic. In 1979 Sones urged Sheldon to contact Grüntzig regarding the possibility of his moving to Cleveland and joining the Department. On the evening of Thursday August 9, 1979, Sheldon met with Grüntzig and his wife Michaela in the cocktail lounge of the Miami Airport Hotel to discuss their coming to Cleveland. A few days later Grüntzig called him from Zurich. Although Michaela was reluctant to move so far away, they were definitely interested if a permanent visa could be obtained. They met again on November 13, 1979 at the American Heart meeting in Anaheim.

In order for the Clinic to initiate the necessary legal measures to obtain a permanent visa for Grüntzig he had to be officially appointed to the Staff. This was done, and we set about obtaining the supporting letters from dozens of leading cardiologists in the U.S.A. that Grüntzig was well trained and held unique skills that would benefit this country. This effort was successful and Grüntzig was exempted from the Visa Qualifying Examination. Meanwhile however, in Atlanta, Robert Woodruff, the long-time CEO of the Coca Cola Corporation had donated $100 million to Emory University Medical School, then the largest ever single contribution to a medical school. Dr. J. Willis Hurst of Emory, unaware of our efforts, contacted Grüntzig about joining the faculty there. Hurst was able to offer Grüntzig two things that we were not: virtually unlimited funds to build a new laboratory dedicated to angioplasty procedures, and a university faculty appointment. Hurst also had better political connections than we did and had no difficulty on obtaining an H-1 visa for him. Grüntzig joined Emory's Department of Cardiology in September 1980.

The first angioplasty at the Clinic was performed in December 1980 by Daniel Phillips. Five years later, on October 27, 1985, Grüntzig and his second wife, Margaret, were killed in a light airplane crash while returning from their island retreat off the coast of Georgia. Those five years were pivotal for Grüntzig, for Emory, and for American cardiology. As he established himself at Emory Grüntzig continued to present annual demonstration courses in coronary angioplasty. Many innovative interventional cardiologists were spawned, and coronary angioplasty became a major industry. Grüntzig, always conservative, decried the aggressive approach to multivessel angioplasty that was espoused by some of those he trained, and he was hesitant to use angioplasty in acute myocardial infarction which others were promoting. Cardiac surgeons began to witness a decline in referrals, except for complications of angioplasty.

In the same year, 1985, Charles Dotter, Melvin Judkins, and Mason Sones also died and America had lost four giants in Cardiology.

In 1978 Loop and the Department of Thoracic and Cardiovascular Surgery learned that the number of fellowship positions approved by the Liaison Committee for Graduate Medical Education would be sharply reduced. They would no longer be able to assign surgical fellows to cover their hospital services and asked for Cardiology's help by expanding hospital coverage by fellows. Since 1975 Cardiology had been attempting to reduce the number of its own fellows and began employing nurses as Departmental Assistants in the catheterization laboratory. We did not have enough fellows available in the Hospital to increase coverage for surgical patients but we found that additional fellows could be provided by reassigning those who were covering the outpatient departments at F-15 and F-25. To facilitate this, for the first time at the Clinic, six individuals trained as physician assistants were employed and trained to take medical histories and perform physical examinations on outpatients. They were given the title of Departmental Assistant IV, mentored by James Hodgman and Daniel Phillips. This proved to be a highly successful program. Many of these individuals subsequently obtained RN degrees and continue to work at the Clinic as nurse clinicians, in the hospital and outpatient department.

After a distinguished career of more than thirty-three years Proudfit retired from clinical practice in December 1979 and was appointed to the Clinical Emeritus Staff as a Senior Consultant. In this capacity he continued to serve as a mentor to Cardiology staff and fellows, he continued his medical research and writing, provided guidance and support for the CVIR, and helped read ECG's. He retired completely in December 1985, but from his home he characteristically continued to do research, collaborate and co-author papers with his colleagues, write on the history of cardiology, and provide manuscript reviews for leading medical journals.

Staff additions in 1978-1980 included Harry Lever (1978) and Donald Underwood (1980) in the Section of Clinical Cardiology at F-15, and Robert Hobbs (1979) in the Section of Cardiac Catheterization at F-25. (Mentioned previously were Victor Morant (1976) in Pacemakers and Electrophysiology, and Douglas Moodie (1978) in Pediatric Cardiology.)

Harry Lever was a graduate of the University of Pittsburgh and the University of Rochester cardiology training program and was a faculty member at the University of Pittsburgh and Director of the Echocardiography Laboratory at Montefiore Hospital. A quiet and unassuming but solid clinician, he joined Salcedo's Cardiac Function Laboratory and became interested in idiopathic hypertrophic subaortic stenosis (IHSS). Working with Bernadine Healy in the 1980s he characterized the different types of IHSS, and has collaborated extensively with surgical and invasive colleagues on results of surgical treatment and alcohol septal ablation for IHSS.

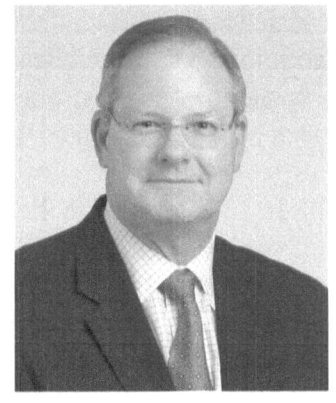

Donald A. Underwood

Donald Underwood graduated from Case Western Reserve University School of Medicine and was a fellow in Clinical Cardiology at the Clinic. He was a quiet, soft spoken clinician who became skilled in ECG interpretation under Proudfit and Lewis and a popular consultant within the Department. He played a key role in the development of radionuclear-stress tests in the Function Laboratory and Nuclear Cardiology. Underwood was also an outstanding teacher, and became leader of the

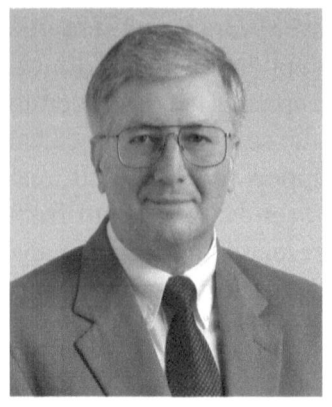

Robert E. Hobbs

medical student educational program that began in 1977. He would later become the Head of the Electrocardiography Section. Hobbs was a native Pennsylvanian, a graduate of Thomas Jefferson University, also trained at the clinic, and was a talented teacher. For many years as a member of the Education Committee he coordinated the training program for internal medicine rotating fellows. He became interested in heart failure and collaborated with cardiac surgeons in the medical management and followup of cardiac transplant patients. He established a clinic for heart failure and transplant patients. [13] Earlier appointees Ravi Rao left in 1975 to join Joel Webster in private practice in Charlotte, North Carolina, Augusto Pichard left in 1975 to join the Washington Cardiology Center in Washington DC, and Hector Lardani left in 1977 to return to his native Buenos Aires, Argentina.

The Century Project Launched

Other clinical departments began to outgrow the main Clinic building, and by now the hospital was again at capacity. After obtaining a certificate-of-need from Ohio authorities in 1979 for additional hospital beds the Clinic began to plan for a new outpatient building on East 100th Street and a further expansion of hospital facilities. The new outpatient building would include satellite cardiology testing facilities to serve clinical departments located there: ECG, ECG stress testing, and echocardiography. The hospital addition would include additional cath labs, new operating rooms, and expanded office and outpatient facilities for the cardiovascular services. This became known as the Century Project.

In 1979 Loop and colleagues began a blood conservation program to reduce the requirement for transfusions during open heart surgery through collection of blood during induction of anesthesia and autotransfusion of this and blood harvested intraoperatively at the end of the procedure. Leonard Golding, a member of Thoracic and Cardiovascular Surgery since 1976 began studies of a left ventricular assist device in patients with advanced cardiac failure.

By 1980 the Cardiology staff had grown to 21 members, plus Sones and Proudfit as Emeritus Consultants. The effects of the VA Cooperative Study had dissipated and clinical activities in Cardiology and Cardiac Surgery were again at record levels with more than 19,000 outpatient visits, nearly 6000 cardiac catheterizations, 4000 echocardiograms, over 800 permanent pacemaker insertions and electrophysiologic studies, and 3200 open heart procedures. The waiting list for catheterizations had reached 520, and for surgery, 200. Increasing numbers of catheterization patients were done "TCI" (to-come-in, i.e. admitted as hospital patients on the day of the procedure and not the day before, as had been routine); some of these patients were discharged to the hotel a few hours after their catheterization. Outpatient catheterizations, the logical extension, began in 1981. [14] Soon Cardiac Surgery arranged for the preoperative workup of elective surgery patients prior to admission, admitting them to the hospital on the day of surgery. (As the planning for the Century Project continued, Sheldon, in 1983, informally proposed that the three cardiovascular services become organized as a cardiovascular division. However this was too revolutionary and politically charged; neither Clinic leadership nor the other cardiovascular department chairmen were ready to consider such a reorganization.) [15]

Until now adult catheterizations had been done only from brachial artery cutdowns. In 1980 Robert Hobbs and Khosrow Dorosti visited several other centers to acquire experience with the Seldinger technique via the femoral artery that Judkins used. It was felt that this would be important to include in the training program for invasive fellows. Gradually, as others also learned this approach, it was employed more frequently. Over the course of the next fifteen years it became the preferred approach by most Clinic angiographers.

After the demonstration that intravenous thrombolytic therapy increased survival in patients with acute myocardial infarction,[17] and intracoronary streptokinase held promise if administered early in the course of acute myocardial infarction,[18-20] we began to plan an emergency triage program for patients with acute myocardial infarction for either intravenous or intracoronary streptokinase, and possible surgical intervention if a residual lesion persisted. [16]

In 1979, Heupler and Hart became Co-Chairmen of the Education Committee succeeding Razavi. The number of fellows had been reduced from 42 in 1975 to 30 in 1980, and the proportion of foreign graduates in the training program was reduced by half. In 1981 the number of internal medicine fellows assigned for rotations in Cardiology was reduced which imposed an additional burden upon cardiology fellows for night and weekend on-call duty. A "moonlighting" program was inaugurated in which cardiology fellows would be able to volunteer as paid "moonlighters" to provide coverage for cardiology patients in the hospital, reducing the need for internal medicine fellows and supplementing the usual on-call coverage by first year fellows. This had the additional advantage making more experienced second and third year cardiology fellows available to aid and consult with first year fellows and the few remaining internal medicine rotators on difficult patients.

Also in 1981 the invasive track of the training program was increased from two to three years and broadened to accommodate training experiences in new programs and procedures that had recently been introduced (in addition to training in cardiac catheterization, ECG and hospital rotations): echocardiography, stress testing and nuclear studies, pacemakers and electrophysiology, Holter testing and the Arrhythmia Clinic, and Pediatric Cardiology. In addition, a "research module" was included in the rotations for all Cardiology fellows, and each fellow was expected to complete a research project or clinical investigation in the course of his training. These projects would be presented to Staff and fellows at a special Fellows' Research Day seminar in the spring before graduation. The first of these would be held in 1983 and the author of the best project would be awarded a prize.

In the fall of 1981 Sones was discovered to have a pulmonary lesion that proved to be a bronchogenic carcinoma for which he underwent surgical resection which was considered successful—the lesion was well encapsulated and there was no sign of metastases. He returned to his work, his busy referral practice, catheterizations, a busy speaking schedule, and the SCAI. Conrad Simpfendorfer, a Chilean native who had graduated from the invasive training program at the Clinic and returned to his homeland in 1979, returned to the Clinic in 1980 as a Clinical Associate in Cardiology and covered Sones' practice when he was away. Simpfendorfer joined the Staff in 1982. He soon became interested in interventional cardiology, and later took on the responsibility for the PTCA Registry. In about 1982 Sones became aware of his declining skills in the laboratory and turned over his catheterization practice to Simpfendorfer. He remained on the Staff and continued to be involved with new technology in the Catheterization Laboratory.

In 1981 James Maloney, a Mayo trained electrophysiologist, was appointed to the staff in the Section of Pacemakers and Electrophysiology, and he became Director of the Electrophysiology Laboratories the following year. Later he would become President of NASPE, the North American Society for Pacing and Electrophysiology (1990). In 1982 Richard Sterba, a Duke trained pediatric cardiologist joined Moodie in Pediatric Cardiology, and a Pediatric Outreach program was launched. Sterba had special expertise in arrhythmias and electrophysiological problems in infants and children and worked also in the Pacemaker/EP Section. Daniel Phillips became Director of Interventional Angiography in the Section of the Cardiac Catheterization Laboratory.

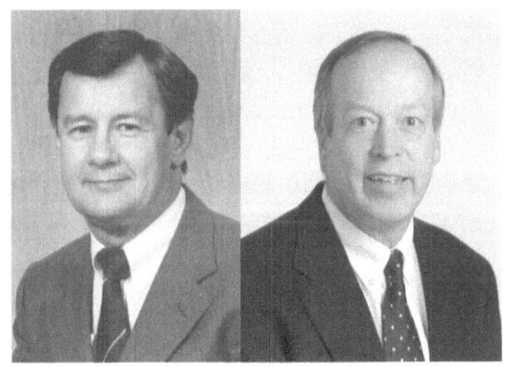

James A. Maloney   Richard Sterba

Building on the success of nurses as assistants in the catheterization laboratories (Departmental Assistant-III's), a nurse-clinician program was launched in 1982 to assist staff members with hospital coverage, along with the Departmental Assistant IV's (physician assistants). This proved to be highly popular as these nurses could be permanently assigned to one or two physicians becoming familiar with their patients, lightening the duties of fellows, and helping also in the outpatient department. There was an advantage also in that these nurses were more or less permanently assigned, and did not rotate off the service as did fellows each module. Moreover they were available to help in the outpatient department.

Hart left for private practice in Pittsburgh in 1982 and Salcedo replaced him as Co-Chairman of the Education Committee.

In the fall of 1982 Andreas Grüntzig called with a recommendation. Jay Hollman had been his first fellow after he started at Emory in September 1980, and impressed him with his skill and intellect. Grüntzig felt somewhat obligated to the Clinic after defaulting on his commitment to join our Staff, and believed that Hollman could become a leader in coronary angioplasty. Phillips had been named Director of Interventional Cardiology in 1982, and by the end of that year Phillips and Heupler had performed 155 angioplasties and others were becoming interested. Hollman joined the staff in January 1983 and proved to be a skillful and aggressive interventionist. It was not long before Dorosti and Franco also learned angioplasty and became interventional angiographers, as later did Conrad Simpfendorfer. In 1983 Hollman, Phillips and Franco performed 507 percutaneous angioplasties. Phillips, however, left for private practice in Pensacola Florida in July 1983, and Hollman succeeded him as Director of Interventional Angiography. Adnan Zaidi was appointed the first special fellow in interventional cardiology.

John Kramer, who had joined the Staff in the Catheterization Laboratory in 1975, became interested in laser applications in cardiac catheterization. In 1982 he embarked upon a joint venture with scientists at the Massachusetts Institute of Technology, Michael Feld and others. Room 4-A of the cardiac catheterization laboratory was commissioned in 1983 as a Laser Research Laboratory. There began a highly fruitful program and the MIT-Cleveland Clinic team learned about lasers of different wavelengths, the difficulties in creating steerable laser catheters, and the role laser spectroscopy and laser induced fluorescence played in analyzing coronary intimal tissue, and treating arteriosclerotic plaques.

Sones announced that he would retire on December 31, 1983. In November he received the Lasker Award, and a Special Symposium honoring Sones was held on November 12, 1983, with a distinguished international faculty. That evening, at a gala testimonial dinner, it was announced that the cardiac catheterization laboratories in a new expanded cath lab area, part of the Century construction project, would be designated the Sones Cardiac Catheterization Laboratories.

The Cost Containment Era

1984 brought substantial changes in the practice of medicine when cost-plus reimbursement for health care was replaced with prospective fee schedules for diagnosis related groups (DRG's). The Clinic was deeply into the Century project, which involved construction of a new outpatient building, the "A Building" (later Crile Building), a new hospital tower, new cardiothoracic operating rooms, expanded catheterization stress, and echo laboratories, and additional cardiovascular offices and outpatient facilities. Training cardiologists and cardiac surgeons had populated competing centers throughout Ohio, and the Clinic's "share" of cardiovascular procedures in Ohio began to fall. As net revenue fell below projections, the cardiovascular departments were closely scrutinized and mixed messages emanated from Clinic administration. General clinical cardiologists, sought to provide referrals to procedurally oriented cardiologists and surgeons, were in short supply as trainees increasingly gravitated toward interventional, imaging, and electrophysiological subspecialties. Cardiologists were beginning to seek "protected time" to pursue their growing research interests, salaries were restrained, and discontent was emerging within the Department.

Still cardiovascular activities were expanding. Intraoperative electrophysiology procedures began in 1983 with ventricular mapping. Intraoperative insertion of automatic internal cardioverter devices began shortly thereafter. The first cardiac transplant since the abortive effort of 1968 was performed in 1984 by Robert Stewart and a transplant coordinating committee was formed. It was not long before the Clinic became one of top three centers in the country for cardiac transplantation. Doppler imaging was introduced in the echocardiograph laboratories (as well as intraoperative Doppler in the operating rooms). Within two years virtually all ultrasound studies would be echo-Doppler studies. In 1980-1986 digital subtraction angiography (DSA) (as applied to coronary and carotid angiography and intravenous ventriculography) was explored in the cath lab with prototype equipment on loan from Philips Medical Systems Inc.[21] Dr. John Yiannikas, a special fellow in imaging, working with Moodie and others studied its use in patients with congenital heart disease. Earlier, Clinic radiologists had touted cut-film DSA as an alternative to coronary arteriography. The equipment was expensive, and satisfactory images required prolonged breath-holding, and as additional space was needed for other emerging digital applications in the cath labs, DSA died a natural death.

In 1984 an Interventional Cardiology track, a four-year program, was added to the training programs. By 1984 the problem of post-angioplasty restenosis had become apparent. Shirey began to explore the use of a temperature sensitive metal coil as a possible stent to maintain lumen integrity after coronary angioplasty. Two years later Hollman was investigating the use of nitinol stents in rabbit and canine models.

William Stewart, a graduate of Harvard and the University of Cincinnati and trained in echocardiography at the Massachusetts General Hospital, and William Schiavone, a graduate of the Clinic's Cardiology program joined the staff in the Cardiac Function Laboratory in 1984 and introduced Doppler echocardiography. [17] With the addition of Gordon Blackburn PhD as a clinical associate in 1985, a Canadian with a PhD in exercise physiology from the University of Pennsylvania, plans were initiated for a cardiovascular rehabilitation program.

An ECG outreach program was launched offering computerized ECG interpretation to nearby hospitals and a Holter scanning service was initiated for outside physicians. A task force to develop a comprehensive computerization program in Cardiology was established under Douglas Moodie. This was envisioned to include: a cardiology information network, a core patient demographic database, a word processing/office management system, computerized Echo data and reports, a stress lab reporting system, cath lab data management, EP data management, a Pacemaker Registry, and a PTCA Registry. [18]

Phase I of the Century construction project was completed in 1985. This included the "A" Building, later named the Crile Building, and one of two planned new interventional laboratories in the Hospital Cath Labs (Room 7; Room 8 would not be completed until 1989). A Cardiology satellite in the "A" building included ECG, echocardiogram, stress testing and office facilities for consultations serving the other departments located in the "A" building. Clinical cardiologists covered these services on a rotating schedule. The training programs were broadened to include a three-year track in Pacemakers and Electrophysiology. Shirey turned over the directorship of the cardiac catheterization laboratories to Fred Heupler, although he continued to perform catheterizations until he retired in 1988. Heupler and Salcedo relinquished their co-chairmanship of the Education

Committee to Donald Underwood and Robert Hobbs. Frank Petrovic became fiscal coordinator for Cardiology.

In early 1984 Shirey had been informed by John Florio that the coronary arteriogram that he was next scheduled to do would be the 100,000th such study in the laboratory. Sones had stopped working in the laboratory about a year earlier. In March of that year Sones and Shirey were each given Golden Catheter Awards by USCI in recognition of their pioneering work. As previously noted a recurrence of bronchogenic carcinoma—or a new primary—was discovered in 1984 for which Sones underwent radiation therapy. In March 1985 Philips presented to the Clinic a contribution of $1 million in equipment for the Sones Laboratories. Shirey recalls Sones' last visit to the catheterization laboratory:[22]

> While I was performing a diagnostic study, he suddenly entered the room and approached me at the patient's side. We were, of course, all delighted to see him. With a hug, tears in his eyes and sadness in his voice, he said, "Thank you for the many years we had together!" The atmosphere of surprise and joy in his visit quickly turned to sorrow. A futile attempt to respond in an appropriate manner was interrupted by his departing words, "Promise me one thing. Be sure Gerri and my family get the very best medical care!"

He received the Galen Award in July, and died in August 1985. [19]

In 1986 Philip Currie, an Australian and Mayo trained ultrasonographer, joined the Staff in the Cardiac Function Laboratory, as did Corrine Bott-Silverman and Patrick Whitlow in the Catheterization Laboratory. Bott-Silverman was a product of the Cardiology invasive-track training program, and worked with Kramer in the Laser Research Laboratory.

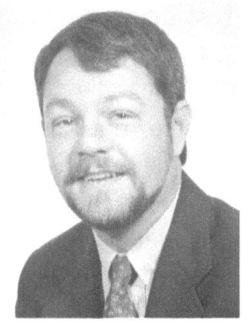

Patrick L. Whitlow

Whitlow was an interventional angiographer from the University of Alabama. He was also appointed Director of the Coronary Intensive Care Unit, succeeding Hodgman.

Fuad Jubran, a CWRU trained cardiologist who came to the Clinic from Lebanon in the Fall of 1986 was a full time assistant in the Coronary Intensive Care Unit playing a key role as a teacher. Royston Lewis turned the directorship of the ECG section over to Donald Underwood. Douglas Moodie was named Chairman of the Department of Pediatrics and Rick Sterba became the head of the Pediatric Cardiology section. Earl Shirey and Royston Lewis retained their directorships of the invasive cardiologists at Desk 25 and clinical cardiologists at Desk 15, and remained co-vice chairmen of the Department.

Floyd Loop had married Bernadine Healy in 1985, a Johns Hopkins graduate and recent Deputy Director of Science and Technology Policy in the Reagan administration. She became Chairman of the Clinic's Research Institute and also a member of the Department of Cardiology. William Stewart assumed the chairmanship of the Cardiology Research Committee and for the first time Cardiology became a participant in multicenter research trials: the Bypass-Angioplasty Revascularization Intervention Trial (BARI),[23-25] and the Bypass Graft Patency Intervention Trial. A Kellogg Foundation multi-center analysis of cost containment in catheterization laboratories also commenced with Fred Heupler as principal investigator. Drs. Salcedo, Robert Tarazi of the Research Division and Ray Go of Nuclear Radiology received a SCORE grant in 1995 to study cardiac function in hypertensive cardiovascular disease.

Also in 1986 Phase II of the Century Project was partly completed including a new Cardiology Appointment Desk, a new Cardiology Testing area including expanded ECG, echo and stress testing facilities, at F-16. In addition Phase II provided additional offices and outpatient facilities at F-15 (Clinical Cardiology) and F-25 (Invasive Cardiology and Cardiac Surgery), and new catheterization waiting and monitoring areas (Desk F-26). In the Hospital the cardiovascular services moved into new facilities on the ninth, tenth, and eleventh floors. The new Coronary Intensive Care Unit was nearby on the second floor, with an angiography-capable special procedure room. The cardiovascular intensive care units were on the third floor next to the Cardiothoracic Anesthesia offices, and the Cardiac Operating Rooms were on the fourth floor, including OR-49, a special operating room that was equipped as a satellite catheterization laboratory for emergent preoperative or intraoperative angiography. [20] All but three floors of the new tower were dedicated for cardiovascular services. [21] Phase III would be completed in 1989 with a second interventional cath lab (Room 8), and three new pacemaker/electrophysiology laboratories (Rooms 9, 10 and 11). Despite this there was continuing concern that there might not be room for continued growth of Cardiology programs and services in existing facilities.

A Phase-I **Cardiac Health Improvement and Rehabilitation Program** ("CHIRP") for postoperative, post-infarction and post-angioplasty patients in the hospital was launched in 1986 with Blackburn and Underwood as Co-Directors, and a new Cardiovascular Screening Center was opened on the first floor of the new hospital building under co-directors Ernesto Salcedo and Herb Naito of the Research Institute. This Center was intended to offer a screening service for families and other visitors, and employees. An Acute Myocardial Infarction Intervention program was launched with a multidisciplinary task force headed by Fred Heupler. Within one year 166 patients with acute coronary syndromes were triaged from 48 regional hospitals.

A third year was added to the noninvasive cardiology training track that would begin in 1988. Now both the invasive and noninvasive programs were three-year programs, with an optional fourth year for those interested in cardiac imaging, interventional cardiology, or cardiac electrophysiology.

In 1987 Tony Simmons, a graduate of Case Western Reserve University and the Clinic's training program in pacemakers and Electrophysiology, and Bruce Wilkoff, also a CWRU graduate with training in electrophysiology and pacemakers at Ohio State University were appointed to the staff in the Section of Pacemakers and Electrophysiology. Fernando Grigera, an Argentinean native, completed an interventional fellowship in 1986 and was offered a staff appointment in 1990 upon completion of visa requirements. In the meanwhile he was accepted as a special fellow in balloon valvuloplasty in the laboratory of Alain Cribier of Rouen, France. The first mitral and aortic balloon valvuloplasties at the Clinic were performed in 1987. Carl Gill left to become Chief Executive Officer of Cleveland Clinic Florida. Robert Stewart filled the gap, and

Eliot Rosenkranz, a pediatric cardiac surgeon joined Cardiac Surgery in 1988. Transesophageal Doppler-echocardiography was explored in the Cardiac Function Laboratory by Drs. Stewart, Schiavone and Currie, and soon this would be extended to the operating rooms where it became indispensable in valve surgery.[26]

Lucile Vanderwyst, who had been head and supervisor of the Cardiac Catheterization Laboratories since 1952 when the first laboratory was started by Sones, retired after 35 years in 1987. Mary Heisler was her successor. Also in 1987 John Florio, Department Administrator, accepted a position as Administrative Director at Cleveland Clinic Florida. Frank Petrovic took over the dual responsibility of Department Administrator as well as Fiscal Coordinator. Margie Horn continued as administrative assistant for the Cardiology Appointment Desk F-14, and Desks 15 and 16.

In 1987 Cardiology initiated a new venture exploring the use of young physicians trained in internal medicine or cardiology as hospital based physicians. These later became known as house physicians or "hospitalists" (Clinical Associates). Under the direction of one or more staff cardiologists these physicians assisted with the care of their hospital patients. They quickly became adept at recognizing problems, initiating emergency treatment when necessary, interfacing with fellows and nurse clinicians, and dealing with sometimes obtuse hospital administrative and nursing issues. Three "hospitalists" were hired in 1987. [22]

The unique status of Cardiology at the Cleveland Clinic was brought into focus by a 1985 survey of 94 academic chiefs of cardiology delineating their rankings for division priorities:

1. Special diagnostic studies
2. Special therapeutic services
3. In-patient consultations
4. Clinical research
5. CCU services
6. Teaching students
7. Training clinical fellows
8. In-patient care
9. Outpatient care

10. Training research fellows
11. Training internal medicine residents
12. Basic science research
13. Continuing medical education
14. Training programs in community hospitals

Their priorities for inpatient and outpatient care were far down the list, and none gave any priority for preoperative or postoperative surgical support.

Russell Raymond, a graduate of the interventional training program, joined the Staff in 1988, and Fuad Jubran was advanced to Staff in Clinical Cardiology where he became Assistant Director of the Coronary Intensive Care Unit. Bill Schiavone left for private practice with a group of former Cardiology fellows in Akron, Ohio. Earl Shirey announced his plans for retirement at the end of the year, although he would continue on a part time basis as an Emeritus Consultant, teaching, doing outside film reviews for Cardiac Surgery, and teaching in the cath lab.

Bruce Wilkoff took over the chairmanship of the Cardiology Information Network Task Force. The computerization project was temporarily stalled pending installation of equipment to be linked with the network in several areas. The **PTCA Registry** was launched under the directorship of Conrad Simpfendorfer.

Cleveland Clinic Florida opened in March 1988, and Tom Noto, a former Cardiology Fellow was appointed to the CCF-Florida Staff. Noto spent several months in Cleveland performing cardiac catheterizations pending approval of his privileges at Broward General Hospital in Fort Lauderdale. [23] Electrocardiograms from CCF Florida were transmitted electronically to the ECG Laboratory for computer assisted interpretation and storage.

The Residency Review Committee of the Liaison Committee for Graduate Medical Education ordered that on-call time for residents and fellows be limited. Suddenly all institutions, even academic centers, began to compete for "moonlighters" to supplement night and weekend coverage in hospitals. Moonlighting was not considered in the formula for calculating on-call time.

The first valvuloplasty was performed in the Cath Lab in January 1987, the first coronary atherectomy in August, 1988. Peripheral vascular angioplasties were also performed in the cath lab for the first time in January, 1988. After much discussion, Cardiology agreed to provide a special tutorial for Robert Graor, a member of the Department of Peripheral Vascular Disease, to prepare him for Board Certification in Cardiovascular Disease. Graor had participated in research with recombinant tissue plasminogen activator (tPA) in venous thromboembolism and was interested in expanding this work into arterial thromboembolism, as well as performing peripheral angioplasties independently in the cardiac catheterization laboratory. There was no precedent for a noncardiologist to have privileges in a cardiac catheterization laboratory and Graor intended to become board certified in Cardiovascular Disease, an intent never fulfilled. Several of our interventional cardiologists were also interested in tPA and the possibility of doing peripheral vascular interventions.

In 1989 Cardiology and Peripheral Vascular Disease began to plan for a peripheral vascular laboratory adjacent to but part of the cardiac catheterization laboratory complex. Graor had obtained partial funding for equipment. However Radiology and Vascular Surgery opposed the concept until all agreed that radiologists and vascular surgeons who were appropriately trained in peripheral vascular interventions would also have access to the laboratory. Angiographic equipment was surveyed and bids were solicited. After some misadventure into the bidding process by a staff member, construction of the laboratory was completed and Philips angiographic equipment was installed in Room 12 of the Cardiac Catheterization Laboratories in 1991. [24]

Cost Containment and the McKinsey Plan for Cardiology

1988 witnessed a sobering reality of the economic crisis that was occurring in the health care industry. Rising costs, limited reimbursement by Medicare and other third party providers, together with pressures imposed from competition and grossly overestimated expectations for the newly opened Cleveland Clinic Florida, all caused Clinic administration to embark upon a radical cost containment strategy. The McKinsey Company was hired to help develop a comprehensive financial stabilization plan. Expenditures were curtailed, capital equipment requests were cancelled, staff salaries were capped, and employee structure adjustments were frozen. All departments were called upon to reduce their employee complements. For several years Cardiology had provided matching funds from its endowment to support Research-Review-Committee-approved clinical research projects. [25] Although it had never been intended to be a profit center, it became necessary to close the Cardiovascular Screening Clinic. The professional staff became increasingly disenchanted, even cynical, and began to scrutinize Clinic leadership and their decisions.

In January and February of 1989 two retreats were held by Cardiology in order to address issues of growth, improved efficiency with cost containment, and staff satisfaction. It was concluded that (a) there was potential for continued growth of cardiology productivity although this would require additional staff, (b) all staff should be encouraged to devote a half day each week for research and/or administrative purposes (several had already been authorized to shelter 40-50 percent of their time for research purposes, with Board of Governors encouragement), and the coverage to make this possible should be provided by physician clusters within each Section, (c) Cardiology Staff reaffirmed their commitment to provide facilitated access for surgical patients, (although by this time dissent was emerging among some of the subspecialists in the Department for providing this service to Cardiac Surgery), (d) Cardiology would make a concerted effort to improve access for patients by filling any open appointment slots with new or urgent patients forty-eight hours in advance, (e) McKinsey's proposed concept for "geographic coverage" of patients on various hospital floors was rejected, as was their proposal for routine follow-up of cardiology patients by noncardiologists in other departments, and (f) Foundation leadership needed to be apprised of the opportunities afforded by Cardiology and the need for appropriate resources to realize these opportunities. This led to a special Department Meeting with the Chairman and Vice Chairmen of the Board of Governors on March 14, 1989. Staff concerns were heard, but no commitments for relief were forthcoming.

In 1989 Phil Currie became disenchanted with the atmosphere at the Clinic and resigned to enter private practice. However Paul Casale, a Cornell graduate, joined the Staff as an interventional cardiologist in the Cath Lab Section in 1989, as did Daniel Murphy, a native Californian who trained at

Childrens Hospital in Cincinnati, in Pediatric Cardiology, Richard Trohman, a Michigan Graduate who trained in Clinical Electrophysiology at Jackson Memorial Hospital in Miami, in Pacemakers and Electrophysiology, Alan Klein, a McGill graduate and Mayo trained ultasonographer, in the Cardiac Function Laboratory, and Fred Pashkow in the Cardiac Function Laboratory as Medical Director of the Cardiac Rehabilitation Program (CHIRP).

Phase III of the Century project was finally completed with the construction of the second dedicated interventional laboratory (Room 8) in the Cath Lab, and three new pacemaker/electrophysiology laboratories and adjacent workspace (Rooms 9, 10, 11). The cath lab complex was dedicated as the Sones Cardiac Catheterization Laboratories on October 20, 1989.

Jay Hollman, Director of Interventional Cardiology, proved to be an aggressive protégé of Grüntzig and tackled multivessel lesions, angioplasty in acute myocardial infarction, as well as a few patients in shock, with many notable successes. However, as complications with these patients increased he came under increasing pressure from surgical colleagues to avoid these high-risk cases. Hollman resigned in 1990 and entered private practice in Baton Rouge, LA.

Transition 1

In 1989 the Clinic's financial situation had not improved. The Florida venture had fallen far behind expectations and required large infusions of support from Cleveland. Additional bond issues were floated to provide cash for operations. McKinsey and Company was hired to review and advise the Clinic regarding financial management, organizational structure and governance. William Kiser, Chairman of the Board of Governors came under increasing pressure, and resigned on July 29, 1989. [26]

A search committee consisting of the Board of Governors and members of the Board of Trustees began the process of identifying Kiser's successor. [27] In the meanwhile a transition team headed by Fawzy Estafanous, Chairman of the Division of Anesthesia directed the operations of the Clinic. McKinsey and Company formulated a plan envisioned to provide cash reserves of $60 million after three years with cost containment, improved efficiency and enhanced patient flow. Special task forces were appointed to address the Florida venture, institutional marketing, and resource utilization. An "Activity Value Analysis" (AVA) was initiated for all administrative areas of the Foundation. Physician productivity was scrutinized, and a proposal for "level scheduling" of patients by cardiology physicians was presented, to be applied ultimately in all departments. This required strict time allotments for each new patient, former patient, consults, and procedures. McKinsey also proposed a Continuing Care Clinic for former Cardiology patients to be staffed by internists that was summarily rejected as unpopular with patients and counterproductive. Patient satisfaction in Cardiology had been among the highest throughout the Division of Medicine. McKinsey did not understand the nature of the patient-physician relationship. The effect of these efforts on staff morale was profound.

Transition 2

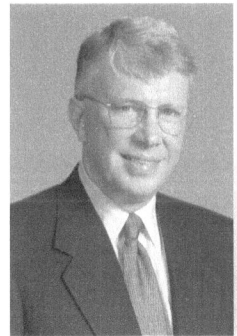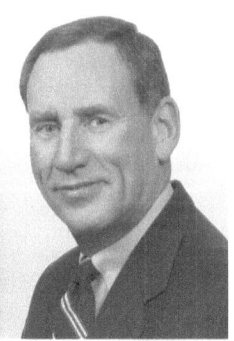

Floyd Loop was named Chairman of the Board of Governors in November 8, 1989, and Delos (Toby) Cosgrove succeeded him as Chairman of the Department of Thoracic and Cardiovascular Surgery. A Massachusetts General Hospital trained surgeon, Cosgrove joined the Clinic In 1975 and had gained national recognition for valve surgery, particularly mitral valve repair.

Floyd D. Loop   Delos M. Cosgrove

The McKinsey project continued throughout 1990. Loop wanted to build new leadership throughout the Foundation and many changes occurred over the next two years when more than 24 department and division chairmen were added or replaced. Kiser retired, Dan Harrington was named Chief Financial Officer replacing Jerry Wolf, John Eversman, Chief Operating Officer, resigned and was replaced by Frank Lordeman, John Clough was named Director of Health Affairs, Rob Kay was named Chief of Medical Operations, and Richard Farmer, Chairman of the Division of Medicine, was replaced by Muzzafar Ahmad. In the course of the Annual Professional

Review of Cardiology in July 1990 Sheldon was advised to step down. He submitted his resignation on August 20, 1990 to become effective as soon as his replacement could be identified, and The Board of Governors appointed a Search Committee for his successor. [28]

Having obtained a permanent visa and completed a traineeship with Alain Cribier of Rouen, France in valvuloplasty, Fernando Grigera returned from Argentina to join the Cath Lab section as an interventional cardiologist in 1990. Tom Marwick, an Australian who had completed a special fellowship in echocardiography was appointed to the Staff in the Cardiac Function Laboratory. [29] Karen James completed invasive cardiology training and a year as Clinical Associate in Electrocardiography, and was appointed to the Assistant Staff in Clinical Cardiology in 1990, later transferring to a new Heart Failure Section. Stress echocardiography was added to the many procedures performed in the Cardiac Function Laboratory. Radiofrequency ablation procedures for ventricular arrhythmias would begin in the EP laboratory in 1991.

In his final Report to the staff in 1990 Sheldon commented:

> I have completed 16 years as Chairman of the Department of Cardiology, and as I dictate this report new leadership is on the horizon. I am proud of what we have accomplished in our Department, and for the Foundation. A comparison of Cardiology activities in 1975 and 1990 is attached. We have participated in, indeed provided the lead for, the greatest growth of the specialty of Cardiovascular Disease in its history. We have expanded the scope of Cardiovascular Disease at the Cleveland Clinic to include virtually all of the subspecialty and technological modalities that are clinically relevant, including Pediatric Cardiology and Cardiac Rehabilitation. We have a breadth of subspecialty interests, as well as depth, although recruitment for Staff in some of the newer technologies has been highly competitive. We have recruited Staff with both procedural and research interests, and in doing so outpatient activity has been diluted. As in all other cardiology programs in this country, physician interest has focused more upon procedures. Despite this, patient activity has increased significantly, and

we continued to provide support to our surgical colleagues that is unparalleled in any other institution in this country. As diagnostic evaluations have shifted from the Hospital to the outpatient department, hospital admissions have not grown as much as outpatient activity but the profile of the hospital patient has become increasingly complex. Despite external restraints on reimbursement, length of stay has increased from 8.2 to 9.3 days.

Cardiology has consistently provided more than half of the Division of Medicine's direct or contributing margin. Cardiology together with Cardiac Surgery (approximately 8% of the CCF Staff) have provided one half of the "direct" margin of the Clinic Division. During the past four years the three cardiovascular Services have contributed half of the "direct" net revenue of the Cleveland Clinic Foundation . . .

It seems unlikely that the expansion of Cardiovascular Disease will continue at the same rate in the 1990's or that the Cleveland Clinic Foundation can continue to depend so heavily on its cardiovascular services. Expanding research initiatives will be necessary to maintain "cutting edge" technology, but this will require new sources of funding. Commitment of Staff to research must be balanced by additional staffing for clinical activity in order to assure continuing access of patients, and the responsiveness to patients and referring physicians that has built our reputation as a Cardiovascular Center of Excellence. If we are to expand research initiatives, so must we also support clinical programs to maintain our position in the competitive marketplace.

This is the challenge for the new leadership. I wish my successor well and stand ready to help him in any way that I can. To my colleagues in the Department, I extend my best wishes, continued friendship, and my sincerest thanks for an exciting and fulfilling 16 years.

Sheldon continued his outpatient and hospital practice, performing cardiac catheterizations for another seven years, retiring completely on December 31, 1997.

Shirey continued as an Emeritus Consultant, teaching cardiology and internal medicine fellows and reviewing outside angiograms for Cardiac Surgery until he fully retired in 1995. He continues to live in Cleveland, enjoys golf, and visits the Clinic regularly.

James Maloney resigned in 1991 moving to the Texas Heart Center in Houston, later returning to Ohio and a practice in cardiac electrophysiology at Timken Mercy Hospital in Canton.

Royston Lewis, who had joined Clinical Cardiology in 1960, was a vice chairman of the new Department of Cardiology, and Head of the Section of Electrocardiography until he retired in 1992. Lewis had an uncanny ability to recall details about his patients and he was known for his wit, proclivity for trivia, and celebration of various Welsh holidays, including St. David's Day. His network for Clinic gossip was unsurpassed. He was a stimulating but benevolent teacher, and his ECG conferences were legendary. He also was a heavy smoker, and despite the Clinic-wide smoking ban that was imposed in the mid 1970s he continued to smoke secretly in his office, his cigarettes and ashtray hidden in his top desk-drawer. After he retired in 1992 his health deteriorated, and he died ten years later—followed in three years by his wife, Sheila.

Fernando Grigera left the Clinic in January 1992 for private practice with a group of former cardiology fellows in Ravenna, Ohio.

Juan Lim retired in 1992, and continues to live in the Cleveland area.

Tony Simmons left in 1992 for Wake Forest University—Bowman Gray School of Medicine where he continues his work in cardiac arrhythmias, pacemakers and electrophysiology as an Associate Professor of Medicine.

Ernesto Salcedo resigned in December 1992 to join a group practice near Jacksonville Florida where be built a substantial group in cardiac imaging. After several years he left for a sabbatical in Saudi Arabia, and currently lives in Denver, Colorado where he is Associate Professor of Medicine and Director of Echocardiography at the University of Colorado.

Paul Casale left in 1993 for private practice in Lancaster, PA. After a brief interval studying in Belgium, Tom Marwick continued in the Cardiac Function Laboratory (later Imaging) until 1998 when he returned to Australia where he has become a prolific researcher in cardiac imaging and stress testing as Professor of Medicine at the University of Queensland in Brisbane.

Lon Castle left in 1994 to join a cardiology group in Elyria, OH, but he later returned and was reappointed in 1998, and continues in the Section of Pacemakers and Electrophysiology working at the Main Campus, and at the Westlake Campus.

Victor Morant suffered a sudden major intracerebral hemorrhage while working in the electrophysiology laboratory one day in May 1998 and retired on disability. He still lives in Cleveland and continues with a rehabilitation program at the Clinic.

Groves retired from the Department of Thoracic and Cardiovascular Surgery in 1983. The next twenty-four years were filled with travel and mountain climbing adventures with his beloved wife, Mary, his skillful woodworking and volunteering at the Holden Arboretum, until he died quietly at 84 in 2007. Taylor retired in 1997, and divides his time between Cleveland and Florida.

The Sheldon years were marked by significant growth in the Department of Cardiology, the emergence of new technology and services, consolidation and strengthening of the cardiology training programs, and development of cardiovascular research. The number of staff physicians in the Department increased from 16 in 1975 to 36 by June 30, 1991. Pacemakers and Electrophysiology and Cardiac Ultrasound, fledgling programs in 1975, became important and sizeable programs by 1991, and Interventional Cardiology emerged as an important new program. Pediatric Cardiology was reintroduced to the Clinic, and Coronary Intensive Care assumed increasing importance as interventional technology brought increasing numbers of patients with acute myocardial infarction to the Clinic. Cardiac rehabilitation was introduced to the Clinic. Outreach programs were established in pediatric cardiology, ECG and Holter monitoring, the latter in the form of computer interpretation and scanning services.

Sheldon managed largely by consensus, and served as the interface between the Department and its Sections and the Division of Medicine and Board of Governors. Staff recruitment was an open process in which all Staff members were encouraged to participate. Most major decisions were reached as the result of discussions at Department meetings and retreats. Section Heads were given unfettered support. Individual Staff members were encouraged do develop their interests in teaching or research, but all were expected to excel in clinical care—but few could be expected to become "triple threats" and excel in all three areas.

Support for Cardiac Surgery grew as an even larger proportion of patients were referred from outside cardiologists with coronary arteriograms performed elsewhere. Cardiology took an even greater responsibility for the postoperative management of surgical patients, and their subsequent followup. Valve surgery was enhanced with intraoperative transesophageal ultrasound, and cardiac transplant surgery was supported by a cardiology team skilled in the management of heart failure. Surgery for cardiac arrhythmias—WPW, atrial fibrillation—was supported by the pacemaker-electrophysiology group that would soon perform ablations in the laboratory. Despite this, under Loop the Department of Thoracic and Cardiovascular surgery distanced itself somewhat from Cardiology, especially as percutaneous coronary angioplasty became widely accepted as an alternative to bypass surgery, nationally as well as locally. (As noted above, even some within Cardiology even questioned the value of this procedure). As cardiology practices became more specialized some became notably disinterested in providing preoperative evaluation, screening and postoperative cardiac care of surgical patients.

The number of fellows in cardiology training programs grew modestly from 42 first and second year fellows in 1975 to 45 in 1991, (the latter includes third year fellows, and fourth year EP, interventional and advanced imaging fellows, as subspecialty programs were introduced); the Clinic's Cardiology Training Program now was the fourth largest in America (after Baylor, Duke, and Johns Hopkins). The addition of paramedical personnel—physicians' assistants, nurse clinicians in the cath labs and in the hospital, and house physicians (hospitalists)—permitted more efficient assignment of fellows, fewer service-related duties, and a better training experience without compromising patient care. This deployment of new kinds of support personnel, medical and paramedical, was new to the Clinic outside of Cardiac Surgery. New training programs emerged—interventional cardiology, and advanced programs in pacemakers and electrophysiology and cardiac imaging. Traineeships for medical students were introduced. Cardiology training for Internal Medicine Fellows never achieved complete success, probably because the technology-related practice of cardiology overshadowed the more academic aspects, as has been a continuing problem with general internal medicine training in an environment dominated by subspecialties.

A great many postgraduate courses and symposia were sponsored by the Department during these years, and hundreds of distinguished national and international speakers and visiting professors participated at Cardiology programs.

The Research Division had traditionally served as the Clinic's primary focus for research. [30] It was not until the late 1970's when research in clinical departments was actually encouraged, and recognized in the process of the annual professional review for staff. Until then clinical research was an after-hours hobby for interested physicians, and many made significant contributions over the years. In the 1970s clinical research grew in importance nationally as the Food and Drug Administration began to require proof of efficacy for new drugs through clinical trials, and multicenter trials emerged, particularly for chemotherapeutic agents. In 1977 the growing popularity of coronary artery bypass surgery stimulated the first major randomized clinical trial in cardiology, the VA Cooperative Study. There was growing support of research by government through NIH grants, and by industry. Clinical and basic research became a more important component of medical school budgets and faculty members became caught up in the "publish or perish" ethic. Universities and medical schools began to publicize their ranking in NIH grants as a means of attracting more research money. Research funds became an important source for not only research, but salaries and operations. Professional grant writers appeared, as did independent, for-profit commercial research organizations. Institutional Review Boards became a necessity to assure patient safety. Hospitals and medical schools began to apply business models to their research endeavors, and the creation of research infrastructures.

On at least two occasions the Board of Governors had considered the possibility of forming a new medical school. The Mayo Clinic had formed a medical school in the early 1970s at least partly to position itself more favorably for NIH grants. John S. Millis, former Chancellor of Case Western Reserve University was the Clinic's consultant in the more recent study, in the mid 1970s. Both times the decision was against forming a new medical school. The Clinic had not yet taken the step of a medical school affiliation but as new staff were recruited with research experience from medical school and post-medical school training programs there was not only more interest in research in clinical departments but also in academic affiliations.

In 1975 cardiology staff members listed 35 ongoing research projects and 26 publications for the year. Although randomized clinical trials were controversial (and disdained by Sones after the VA Cooperative Study), encouraged by Bernadine Healy, Cardiology began to participate in these trials in the late 1980s. In 1990 cardiology staff listed 156 research projects, including several NIH funded multicenter studies, and they published 104 book chapters, papers and abstracts. Many staff members actually had protected research time sanctioned by the Department and the Clinic. Research by fellows was encouraged, and the Department supported this with its endowment funds and by contributions from industry. But what was lacking was a strong research infrastructure for writing grant proposals, organized recruitment of outside funding, support personnel, statistical support, manuscript preparation, and space.

In the 1970's some departments adopted the practice of creating a hospital service in which their hospital patients were managed by one or more physicians on a rotating basis, allowing their colleagues to cover the outpatient department, that seemed more efficient. This "split-service" concept had first been used by the Department of General Internal

Medicine, and was followed shortly thereafter by Hypertension and Nephrology. Initially this concept was decried by cardiologists as not conducive to individualized patient care. Historically cardiologists were responsible for their own patients in the hospital, except when Sones was banned from the hospital other staff members covered his hospital patients. All staff shared in the responsibility for evaluating "mail order" surgical patients and covering them in the hospital. However with the emergence of interventional, electrophysiology and imaging sections—and growing research activities—sections began to organize into "split services," allowing staff to share the coverage of hospital patients on a rotating basis. This had the additional benefit of providing "sheltered" or "protected time" for other activities: outpatients, laboratory procedures, and research. Moreover, educational opportunities were enhanced for fellows who rotated through these hospital services. Soon there were interventional, valve, arrhythmia and surgical services in the hospital, much like the coronary intensive care service. The tradeoff however was that once patients were discharged from the hospital they were less certain of who their cardiologist was, and who would be responsible for their continuing care. Indeed some cardiologists became disinclined to accept a continuing care responsibility in the outpatient department. Arrhythmia clinics, pacemaker clinics, and valve clinics followed, also covered by rotating Section members, further allowing individual staff members to devote more time to procedural and research interests. Patient care indeed became less personalized.

Cardiology facilities were increased substantially with completion of the Century project, but since 1974 each new facility that had been created was filled nearly to capacity within a few years after completion.

With staff growth, and subspecialization within the Department, the intimate social events, and impromptu lunch room conversations were gone and collegiality somewhat diminished, despite more staff participation in planning and governance, regular department meetings and retreats, fellows' picnics and graduation dinners, and departmental Christmas parties. But staff loyalty and commitment to the Clinic has never waned. Most have felt that the type of group practice embodied by the Clinic is without peer.

Notes to The Sheldon Years

1. In designing the outpatient department, Proudfit was to supervise the planning of the first floor, and Sones the second floor. Proudfit had specified examining rooms of a minimum of 120 sq. ft. in size. But in order to fit the specified number of examining rooms into the footprint of the facility the architects had to reduce their size to 80 sq. ft., uncomfortably small for efficient utilization, unbeknownst to Proudfit or Sones until construction was almost complete. The same was true for the both floors. Sones was furious and insisted that the rooms on the second floor be modified creating two-room examining suites, one room for the examining equipment and furniture, and the other was more office-like for patient interviews, writing and consulting. Further, Proudfit and Sones agreed that the construction should provide for possible additional floors to the building to allow for expansion; later it became apparent that the foundation would *not* support additional floors.

2. When Sones moved into his new office that was adjacent to Room 4 of the cardiac cath lab, he learned that electrical interference from the laboratory interfered with his dictating equipment. He was forced to create a new office in an alcove adjacent to the fellows' work area ("bullpen") next to the cath lab complex.

3. Four of these laboratories were "carousel" type laboratories: a preparation room and a post-procedure room were adjacent to each procedure room, so that the time between cases and clean up time could be minimized, increasing "throughput."

4. I believe Cardiology was the first department to produce detailed annual reports. These were also delivered to the Board of Governors to aid in each year's Annual Departmental Review.

5. It was the antithesis of Sones' management style, and more structured than Proudfit's, although some later decried the bureaucratic committee structure within the Department.

6. Additional grants were received from the Saudi Arabian government of $60,000 in October 1975, and $1 million in 1980. Methodist Hospital in Houston had developed a substantial international referral practice in the 1960s, but had done little as an institution to promote it.

7. Mrs. Pat Spaeth was the first Director of the International Center. Arabic, Turkish and Spanish interpreters were hired. Mr. Ben Hosler, then Head of the Clinic's Security Services was key in providing transportation and other support for visiting patients and dignitaries. In about 1980 Mr. John Hutchins succeeded Spaeth, and was named Executive Director of the International Center. The model has been copied by several other medical centers including Johns Hopkins (to which Hutchins was recruited to launch their program), Mayo Clinic and Massachusetts General Hospital all of whom compete for international referrals.

8. It became the responsibility of cardiologists to review cineangiograms performed elsewhere on these patients, advise the cardiac surgeons of their candidacy for surgery, and if accepted perform their preoperative medical evaluations, participate in their postoperative management and, in many cases, conduct their later postoperative cardiac followup.

9. Later, in 1977, a portion of 7-West was assigned to Cardiology as a Cardiac Step-down unit.

10. Kiser had been named to this position by the Board of Governors in 1969. Wasmuth wanted to strengthen the administrative leadership of the foundation, and also to groom sucessors. The Board and Wasmuth chose Kiser after considering several candidates. Later Wasmuth wanted to further broaden the administrative core and appointed Shattuck Hartwell as Vice Chairman in charge of Professional Affairs, and Kiser became Vice Chairman for Operations. Hartwell's arbitrary appointment was questioned by many staff members. Later a search/review committee was formed for the Director of Professional Affairs and after considering many candidates Hartwell was the nominee and confirmed by the Board.

11. Siegel had become involved in a divorce about the time we moved into the new facilities. He remarried within a few months, but this too ended in divorce after a very short time. Depressed, he decided to abandon Ohio and make a fresh start in Florida.

12. Kaltenbach had visited Sones' laboratory in Cleveland on several occasions in the 1960's and '70's, and was among the first to perform coronary arteriography outside of the United States.

13. In the 1990s I had proposed the creation of a Section of Heart Failure in the Department with Hobbs as its Head, but he repeatedly declined.
14. Later a floor of the new Park Plaza Hotel was dedicated as an observation area for patients having outpatient catheterizations, and staffed with an LPN.
15. Excerpt from a memorandum from Sheldon to William Frazier, Chairman of Cardiology Planning Task Force April 25, 1983:

> . . . A similar reasoning might be applied to the Department of Thoracic and Cardiovascular Surgery, and the Department of Cardiothoracic Anesthesia, both of which are growing larger, and experiencing some tendency for subspecialization. Perhaps a Cardiovascular Division should be considered.
>
> A Cardiovascular Division should not attempt to amalgamate specialties, or confuse established hierarchies of specialty and subspecialty training programs. From the standpoint of coordination of medical activities the three cardiovascular departments are already functioning more or less as a division, although they report through different divisions to the Board of Governors. A permanent chairman of a Cardiovascular Division, subordinating any one specialty to another, would be unworkable, but a chairmanship that would rotate among the chairmen of the three departments with a term of office of one or two years, could be workable, particularly if there are only three departments. With a more direct line of reporting to the Medical Operations Group and Board of Governors our sections heads would play a stronger role in the management of their respective areas of responsibility. Policy decisions would flow from the Board of Governors through the Cardiovascular Division chairman to the department heads and section heads. Business functions would reside in a cardiovascular business manager who would report to the Division chairman and a cardiovascular committee (three department chairmen) on one hand, and the Foundation Operations Group (Fiscal, Human Resources, Operations, etc.) on the other.

Whatever organizational structure emerges, it seems likely that Cardiology and its two sister departments will require a facilitated line of communication with top policy and operational management of the institution, and stronger administrative support and coordination among our departments.

Although these thoughts emerge from a Cardiology work group in addressing issues of organizational structure, they require discussion with Fred Loop and George Estafanous before presenting them to any higher body.

I had previously discussed the idea with Loop and Estafanous over dinner at the Park Plaza Hotel. The response was mixed.

16. Sones, on October 29, 1959, had attempted with intracoronary streptokinase to recanalize an occluded right coronary artery of a 43-year old man with an acute myocardial infarction, without success.
17. William Schiavone visited other centers to become familiar with Doppler. techniques in echocardiography and introduced this technology in the Cardiac Function Laboratory in 1984.
18. A computerized Cardiology patient scheduling system had been in effect since 1978.
19. As noted previously, Dotter, Judkins and Grüntzig died in the same year.
20. This never fulfilled its promise. The bulky X-ray equipment left little room for routine surgery. It was occasionally used as a satellite interventional laboratory, but it was inconvenient for this also.
21. The fifth floor was an equipment floor, the Medical Intensive Care unit was on the sixth floor, a special VIP wing was on the seventh floor next to ophthalmology, and the eighth floor and half of the ninth were general med/surg floors.
22. Gradually Departmental Assistant IV's (physicians' assistants) were phased out. Some obtained RN degrees and became nurse clinicians.

23. Carl Gill became CEO of CC-Florida in 1988. In addition to Noto the first cardiologists on the staff were John Lister, an electrophysiologist who was Chief, and Howard Bush, an invasive cardiologist. Clinic physicians were not welcomed at Broward General, and obtaining privileges was fraught with difficulty. The Clinic finally leased beds from and later bought North Beach Hospital, a few miles away, as a stop-gap measure, although North Beach did not have a certificate-of need—for cardiac surgery. This had to be done at Broward.

24. Graor left the Clinic a short time later.

25. To strengthen Cardiology's endowment and support for research and education, a Fund Development Committee was established in 1998 with Royston Lewis, Chairman.

26. In June 1989 Cleveland Clinic Florida was not performing as expected. Loop had been a member of the Board of Governors since 1988 (and his wife Bernadine Healy was chairman of the Division of Research), and the Board was becoming restless about Florida and the Clinic's financial position and Kiser's leadership. McKinsey had been hired to help identify solutions. Kiser was among a group of Clinic physicians attending an international conference in Spain in June 1989. Upon returning he found that he no longer had the support of the Board.

27. The Trustee representatives on the search committee included Arthur Modell, who by now had become a close friend of Loop. Loop admitted to only casual interest in the chairmanship.

28. This was probably the beginning of a plan envisioned by Loop. In the first two years of his administration 21 department chairmen in the Divisions of Medicine and Surgery were replaced.

29. Marwick was a "Clinical Fellow-B," a designation used for foreign graduates who were not yet qualified for medical licensure in Ohio.

30. A major component of the Clinic's support for the Research Division was with revenue from clinical departments calculated to cover (guarantee) at least the staff salaries so this was not a drain upon external research grants. Inasmuch as the Clinic provided and maintained the facilities, it collected the overhead provided from these grants.

References for The Sheldon Years

1. Porter, ME Teisberg EO: *Redefining Health Care. Creating value-based competition on results*. Chapter 5 pp 167-172, Boston: Harvard Bus Sch Press; 2006.

2. Cosgrove DM, Chavez AM, Gill CC, Golding LA, Lytle BW, Stewart RW, Taylor PC, Loop FD: Mitral valvuloplasty at the Cleveland Clinic Foundation. Cleve Clin J Med. 1988; Jan-Feb;55(1):37-42.

3. Cosgrove DM: Mitral valve repair in patients with elongated chordae tendineae. J Card Surg. 1989; Sep;4(3):247-52.

4. Judkins MP: Selective cinecoronary arteriography. Part I. A percutaneous transfemoral technic. Radiol. 1967;89:815-824.

5. Sones FM: The Society for Cardiac Angiography. Editorial. Cath and Cardio Diagn. 1978;4:233-234.

6. Society for Cardiac Angiography News. The Society for Cardiac Angiography: Its purpose, efforts and goals. Cath and Cardiovasc Diagn. 1981;7:217-224.

7. Murphy ML, Hultgren HN, Detre K et.al.: Treatment of chronic stable angina. A preliminary report of survival data of the randomized Veterans Administration cooperative study. NEJM. 1977;297:621-626.

8. Takaro T, Hultgren H, Lipton M, Detre K and participants in the Veterans Administration Cooperative Study Group: VA Cooperative Randomized Study for Coronary Arterial Occlusive Disease. II. Left main disease. Circulation. 1976; 54(suppl 3):107.

9. VA Coronary Artery Bypass Surgery Cooperative Study Group: Eighteen-year follow-up in VA Cooperative Study of Coronary Artery Bypass Surgery for Stable Angina. Circulation. 1992; 86:121-130.

10. European Coronary Surgery Study Group: Coronary-artery bypass surgery in stable angina pectoris: Survival at two years. Lancet. 1979;1:889-893.

11. Chaitman BR, Fisher LD, Bourassa MG, et al: Effect of coronary bypass surgery on survival patterns in subsets of patients with left main coronary artery disease. Am J Cardiol. 1981;48:765-777.

12. CASS Principal Investigators and their Associates: Coronary Artery Surgery Study (CASS): randomized trials of coronary bypass surgery. Survival data. Circulation. 1983;68:939-950.

13. Sheldon WC, Loop FD, Proudfit WL: A critique of the VA cooperative study. Cleve Clin Q. 1978;45:225-230.

14. Loop FD, Proudfit WL, Sheldon WC: Coronary bypass surgery weighed in the balance. Am J. Cardiol. 1978;42:154-6.

15. Proudfit WL. Coronary-artery bypass surgery. Letter to the Editor. Lancet. 1978; 1:495-496.

16. Grüntzig A: Transluminal dilatation of coronary-artery stenosis. Letter to the Editor. Lancet. 1978;1:263.

17. European Cooperative Study Group: Streptokinase in acute myocardial infarction. N Engl J Med. 1979;301:797-802.

18. Ganz W, Buchbinder N, Marcus H et al: Intracoronary thrombolysis in evolving acute myocardial infarction. Am Heart J. 1981;101:4-13.

19. Rentrop P, Blanke H, Karsch KR, Wiegand V, Kostering H, Rahlf G, Oster H, Leitz K: Reopening of infarct-occluded vessel by transluminal recanalisation and intracoronary streptokinase application. Dtsch Med Wochenschr. 1979;Oct 12;104(41):1438-40.

20. Rentrop P, Blanke H, Karsch KR, Kaiser H, Koestering H, Leitz K: Selective intracoronary thrombolysis in acute myocardial infarction and unstable angina pectoris. Circulation. 1981;63:307-317.

21. Detrano R, Yiannikas J, Simpfendorfer C, Hobbs R, Salcedo E: Exercise digital subtraction ventriculography for the detection of ischemic wall motion abnormalities in patients without myocardial infarction. Br Heart J. 1986;56:131-137.

22. Shirey, EK: Personal communication, October, 2006.

23. Taylor PC. Cosgrove DM. Lytle BW. McCarthy P. Stewart RW. Loop FD: Angioplasty versus coronary artery bypass surgery for multivessel disease—a BARI equivalent study. Journal of Invasive Cardiology. 1994;6(3):99-102.

24. Whitlow PL: The Bypass Angioplasty Revascularization Investigation (BARI) trial: implications for clinical practice. Cleveland Clinic Journal of Medicine. 1997;64(1):17-20.

25. Berger PB. Velianou JL, Aslanidou Vlachos H, Feit F, Jacobs AK, Faxon DP, Attubato M, Keller N, Stadius ML, Weiner BH, Williams DO, Detre KM, BARI Investigators: Survival following coronary angioplasty versus coronary artery bypass surgery in anatomic subsets in which coronary artery bypass surgery improves survival compared with medical therapy. Results from the Bypass Angioplasty Revascularization Investigation (BARI). Journal of the American College of Cardiology. 2001; 38(5):1440-9.

26. Stewart WJ. Gill CG. Currie PJ, Schiavone WA. Salcedo EE, Lytle BW, Golding, LA, Agler DA and Cosgrove DM: Intraoperative Doppler color flow mapping in valve conservation surgery. Circulation. 1986;74:II-145.

27. Kramer JR, Proudfit WL, Loop FD, et al: Late follow-up of 781 patients undergoing percutaneous transluminal coronary angioplasty or coronary artery bypass grafting for an isolated obstruction in the left anterior descending coronary artery. Am Heart J. 1989;118:1144-1153.

THE TOPOL YEARS
1991-2006

Eric J. Topol was a native of New York and graduated from the University of Rochester School of Medicine and Dentistry in 1979. He married Susan Leah Merriman in 1979. He did his internship and a residency in Internal Medicine at University of California—San Francisco School of Medicine. In 1982 he moved to Johns Hopkins in Baltimore for a fellowship in Cardiovascular Medicine, in the course of which he returned to San Francisco, to the San Francisco Heart Institute for a special fellowship in coronary angioplasty in 1984. After completing his Cardiology training at Hopkins he joined the faculty at the University

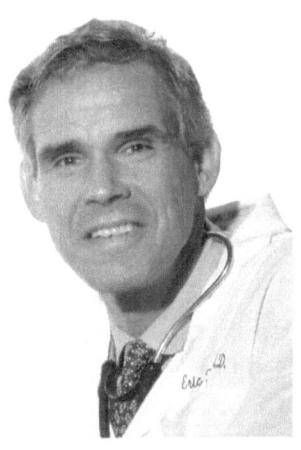

Eric J. Topol

of Michigan in 1985 where he was Associate Director of the cath lab under William O'Neill in Dr. Bertram Pitt's Department of Cardiology. When O'Neill left in 1987, Topol replaced him as Director, and he became a Professor of Medicine in 1990. [1]

Topol first become interested in multicenter clinical trials with Rob Califf of Duke University in the early 1980s. He first met Califf in 1979 as an intern at UC San Francisco, California where Califf was an Assistant Resident. When Califf went to Duke for a fellowship in cardiovascular disease in 1980 they remained good friends. Califf completed his cardiovascular fellowship in 1983, and subsequently became co-director of the Duke Database for Cardiovascular Disease that evolved from a computerized databank that dates to 1968. The first multicenter trial TAMI-1 was started there in 1985. Upon joining the cath lab at the University of Michigan in 1985 Topol led the TAMI 1[1], GUSTO[2] and CAVEAT[3] trials. Thus began a productive collaboration with Rob Califf in many multicenter trials that continues to this date. [2]

In October 1990 he was a candidate to replace Pitt as Chief of Cardiology in Ann Arbor when Muzaffer Ahmad, Chairman of the Clinic's Search Committee for the Chairman of the Department of Cardiology called him and invited him to visit Cleveland. He met the Search Committee and a few Cardiology Staff, and was impressed by the group spirit, the rich heritage, and the excellent clinical reputation of the Department. He felt that it could become an ideal environment in which to conduct clinical trials. During that visit his enthusiasm grew. He excitedly called his wife from the Cleveland airport and told her that this could become their next home.

During his next visit to Cleveland he met Floyd Loop and Bernadine Healy who assured him he would have virtually unlimited support. He accepted the position and was appointed by the Board of Governors on April 17, 1991, arriving in Cleveland in June.

Building a New Department

Topol brought with him several key people from Ann Arbor in 1991. Steve Ellis was an interventional cardiologist whom he had recruited to Michigan in 1986 from Emory University where he had trained under Andreas Grüntzig for a short time before Grüntzig was killed in an airplane crash in 1985. When Topol asked if he would like to join him he accepted without hesitation, although he knew little about the Clinic. He arrived in October and became Director of the Clinic's Catheterization Laboratory. He was already experienced in clinical trials and proved to be an organized administrator and respected mentor in the cath lab.

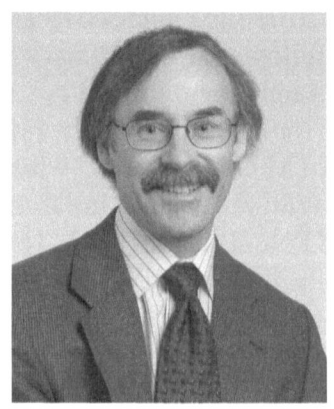

Stephen G. Ellis

Michael Lincoff, a cardiology fellow at the University of Michigan, accompanied Topol as a 3rd year fellow when he came to Cleveland.

Prior to his arrival in Cleveland Topol began a search for new leadership in the Department. He wanted to bring in his own team. He called James Thomas, a rising echocardiographer at the Massachusetts General Hospital, and invited him to look at the Clinic. [3] Thomas had previously turned down an offer from Brigham and Women's Hospital to be head of its echo laboratory.

At about the same time his Angiographic Core Laboratory Director Darrell Debowey attended a meeting in Rotterdam where he heard a lecture by Steve Nissen, then Director of the Coronary Intensive Care Unit at the Hospital of the University of Kentucky, on intravascular ultrasound and was impressed with his presentation. Dobowey mentioned this to Topol, who inquired of Dr. Cindy Grines, then at the University of Michigan, formerly of the University of Kentucky, who had worked with Nissen. Grines gave him a strong recommendation. In the fall of 1991 Topol contacted Nissen, and arranged for him to visit Cleveland.

Thomas and Nissen both visited the Clinic, separately, in 1991. Both were hesitant to leave the university environment, but Topol assured them that with the Clinic's strong clinical program, and the research program that he intended to build, the Clinic would be as good as if not better than any university setting. When they visited they were impressed

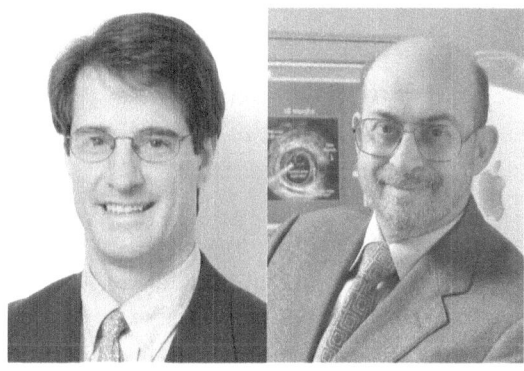

James D. Thomas   Stephen E. Nissen

by Topol's pervasive sense of confidence and enthusiasm, and by the new leadership opportunities offered. Thomas accepted a position as the new Head of Cardiovascular Imaging, and Nissen became Section Head of Clinical Cardiology and Director of the Coronary Intensive Care Unit, both arriving in mid-1992.

Murat Tuzcu, a physician from Turkey, trained in cardiology at the Clinic, and later in interventional cardiology at the Massachusetts General Hospital where he knew both Thomas and Brian Griffin. He returned to join the Clinic Staff in 1992. Tuzcu and Nissen soon joined forces to forge a program in intracoronary ultrasound in the Cath Lab. Thomas was instrumental in susbsequently recruiting Brian Griffin to the staff, and also Pieter Vandervoort and Leonardo Rodriguez, from MGH, to Advanced Imaging fellowships and subsequent staff appointments at the Clinic.

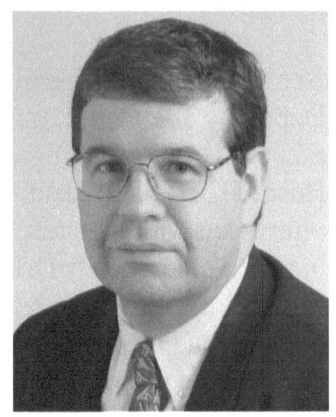

Griffin, a native of Ireland, had met Thomas and Vandervoort, (and also Murat Tuzcu) as a fellow in echocardiography at Massachusetts General Hospital. Upon completion of his training at MGH Griffin accepted a position at Dartmouth's Mary Hitchcock Hospital. Thomas, after joining the Clinic in 1992, encouraged Griffin to join also. At first reluctant to leave Vermont, he visited the Clinic and was impressed with the institution and the people he met including Topol and joined the Staff in February 1993, and Vandervoort joined a short time later.

Brian P. Griffin

Karen James, a Clinical Associate in Clinical Cardiology, was advanced to full Staff in Heart Failure and Transplantation in 1991, and Carol Duffy was appointed to the Staff in Cardiovascular Imaging in 1992. Fetnat Fouad-Tarazi, who had completed a fellowship in cardiovascular disease in the Research Division in 1979, remained on the Staff in that Division where she became interested the neurohumoral control of hypertension and in the problem of syncope. In 1992 she received a dual appointment in cardiology's EP Section where she continues to direct the Syncope Clinic and perform tilt-table testing. Fred Jaeger completed an EP fellowship and joined the Clinical and EP sections as Assistant Staff in 1992, and was advanced to Staff in 1997. He later succeeded Morant as head of the arrhythmia monitoring unit in 1998.

Darrell Debowey, director of Topol's angiographic core laboratory at Michigan, joined him in Cleveland as Director of a new Angiographic Core Laboratory. Valerie Stosic also followed him to become Director of a Clinical Trials Unit to oversee their grants. Both were vital to his ongoing clinical trials: GUSTO, CAVEAT, RESCUE I[4] and EPIC[5]. In addition, Darrel Debowey headed a Graphics and Design laboratory. Loop made available a large unfinished shell space adjacent to the atrium on the first floor of the "G" hospital wing, as well as a string of former anesthesiology offices adjacent to the catheterization laboratories on the second floor, and suddenly the foundations of a research infrastructure were in place. [4] Moreover Topol had broad connections with industry that resulted from his multicenter trials, as a result of which he had no difficulty in attracting generous financial support for his research.

Although Topol had the strong support of Loop and the Board of Governors, his transition to Cleveland was not easy. He was viewed with some skepticism by many in the Department. All previous Cardiology Chairmen had been appointed from within the Clinic. Although it had been the precedent for all prospective members of the Staff to be interviewed by as many members of the Department as possible, many of the Cardiology Staff had never met him. [5] His experience with research and clinical trials was recognized, but Department members took pride in their clinical strengths. The Clinic's cardiovascular reputation was well established. It had ranked No. 2 in the nation by *US News and World Report* in 1990 and No. 3 in 1991. In 1992, shortly after Topol arrived, it was ranked No. 2 again.

Eric Topol was a tall, lean fellow with an awkward smile. He proved to be extremely well organized and was always direct and to-the-point. He had little time for "schmoozing." Some characterized him as "driven" or "single minded." In contrast to Sheldon's style of consensus and participatory management, Topol led by directive, which was not always easily received by older members of the Department. He had a vision of what he wanted the Department to become. He wanted to build a research organization that could thrive on the clinical practice that had been established. Although Section identities were preserved, the committee structure was largely replaced by directors. Steve Nissen was named Vice Chairman of the Department in 1993.

By the end of 1991 the Department was organized clinically into six sections, basically following the preexisting structure with the addition of a Section on Heart Failure and Transplantation.

> The **Invasive Section**, under Steve Ellis included both the clinic
> activities at Desk 25 and the Cath Lab at Desk 26. Pat Whitlow

continued as Director of Interventional Angiography. Mary Heisler continued as Supervisor of the cath lab.

Clinical Cardiology included the clinical activities at Desk 15, the ECG laboratory under Don Underwood, the Coronary Intensive Care Unit under Fuad Jubran, a new Consult Service under Fred Pashkow that would centralize all hospital consultations, and a Surgical Service of willing cardiologists from all sections who would rotate postoperative coverage of unassigned surgical patients.

The Cardiac Function Laboratory became the **Cardiovascular Imaging** Section with Ernesto Salcedo, Director. The Cardiac Health Improvement and Rehabilitation Program continued with Fred Pashkow and Gordon Blackburn, under the combined aegis of Clinical Cardiology and Cardiac Imaging (stress testing). (A Phase II cardiac rehabilitation program was launched in 1991; a cardiovascular screening program was later resurrected as a part of CHIRP in 1989.)

Pediatric Cardiology continued under Rick Sterba, and Pacemakers and Electrophysiology became

Cardiac Pacemakers and Electrophysiology continued under Lon Castle, and Victor Morant continued as Director of Ambulatory Electrocardiography (Holter monitoring and telemetry).

Bob Hobbs headed the new Section of **Heart Failure and Transplantation.**

The **Education Committee** continued initially under Bob Hobbs and Ernesto Salcedo. Although fellows continued the basic rotations, clinic and hospital staff assignments were replaced with section oriented rotations in the hospital, and outpatient clinic assignments, previously deemphasized, were virtually eliminated. Hospital rotations included the Consult Service.

The **Cardiovascular Computing Committee** continued under Bruce Wilkoff.

Within his first two years the research infrastructure that Topol established included:

> Angiography Core Laboratory—Darrell Dobowey, MS
> Cardiology Graphics and Design—Darrell Dobowey, MS
> Cardiovascular Computing Unit—Bruce Wilkoff, MD
> Clinical Trials Unit—Sue Ann Deluca, RN, MS
> Interventional Registry—Jan Howell
> Clinical Investigations (Grant Oversight) Unit—Val Stosik, MBA
> Experimental Interventional Laboratory (1993)—Michael
>   Lincoff, MD

By this time research facilities were becoming scarce. In 1991 the first phase of a massive project to provide expanded research and education facilities was completed with the dedication of the John Sherwin Research Building on the south side of Carnegie Avenue between E 96th and E 100th streets. This plan was the vision of Bernadine Healy, Chairwoman of the Research Institute before she left in May 1991 to become Director of the National Institutes of Health. [6]

The Ohio State Medical School Affiliation

Although the Board of Governors had considered and rejected the idea of a medical school at the Cleveland Clinic on at least two previous occasions, increasing numbers of Clinic Staff members, imbued with the academic ethic, continued to push for a medical school affiliation. Bernadine Healy had laid the groundwork for an affiliation with Ohio State University prior to her departure in May 1991. The liaison was carried on by William Michener and later Andy Fishleder. Medical students from Ohio State would be offered clinical rotations at the Cleveland Clinic. Clinic Staff were offered academic teaching appointments at Ohio State. The agreement was signed in 1991. The clinical rotations began in 1992 and continued for the next ten years, some 30-40 students each year, mainly to primary care services but also to specialty services, including the Cardiology teaching service. The rotations were popular with some Ohio State students, but the Medical School was never very supportive of the affiliation: they did not wish to see their students "farmed-out" to a distant, private teaching facility. Moreover, relatively few Clinic staff applied for formal teaching appointments.

139

As Topol, Ellis, Nissen and Thomas set about organizing the Department and their respective Sections they were confronted by the tradition of staff members each having their own individual practices and referral bases. Although this model had served the Clinic well over the years, it was not the academic model that lent itself to clinical research protocols. Further, none of these new leaders had come from institutions wherein cardiologists had responsibility for postoperative surgical patients. Clearly changes would have to be made. A Consult Service was formed, with rotating staff members assigned to cover cardiology consultations in the hospital. The Imaging Section created rotating teams to cover the outpatient clinic, their hospital patients, hospital consults for echoes and stress tests, and transesophageal echocardiograms in the operating rooms. In the Coronary Intensive Care Unit, coordinated by Nissen, a cardiologist from a rotating group would have total responsibility for patient care replacing the traditional practice of each cardiologist caring for his/her own patients. Soon, two Surgical Services would be formed, with rotating staff cardiologists assigned to cover postoperative patients which their regular cardiologists did not wish to continue while in the hospital.

In the Imaging Laboratory 3-D echocardiography, 4-D tomographic imaging and Contrast echocardiography began to be explored in 1991. In Cardiac Surgery interest in cardiomyoplasty, as a means of improving function of failing hearts, waned after the departure of Roberto Novoa and was replaced by growing interest in the HeartMate left ventricular assist device (LVAD). Intracoronary stents were first used as an adjunct balloon angioplasty in 1991. In the Imaging Section Dobutamine stress echocardiography was explored. The first Restenosis Summit in Cleveland was held on May 28-29, 1992 (No. 4 in a series which Topol had initiated while in Ann Arbor).

Topol continued to recruit aggressively. New Staff additions in 1992 included Gregory Kidwell in Electrophysiology, Tom Karson and Ian Black in Cardiovascular Imaging, and Joseph Sutton in Invasive Cardiology. Edward Plow, formerly at the Scripps Research Institute, was brought to Cleveland to Head the Research Section of the Jacobs Center for Thrombosis and Vascular Biology. [7]

As new staff members were recruited, within the first year six previous Staff members left for various reasons. In 1992 Royston Lewis and Juan Lim retired, Fernando Grigera left for private practice with a group of former Cardiology Fellows in Akron, Ohio, Ernesto Salcedo left for private practice in Florida, Tony Simmons left for private practice in North Carolina, and James Maloney left for Baylor University in Houston. Of twelve new staff additions in 1991 and 1992, five would be gone within six years

The Kaiser Permanente Affiliation

In 1992 Loop signed an agreement with Kaiser Permanente that would allow them to use the Cleveland Clinic Hospital for their patients. As a part of this agreement Kaiser physicians would also have access to our Cardiac Catheterization Laboratories. One had cath privileges in 1992, and this number grew to five by 1996.

Ian Black, a young Australian cardiologist and an Advanced Imaging fellow replaced Hobbs as Director of the Education and Fellowship Program in July 1992. The Education Committee was deemphasized as Topol and Black began to make most of the decisions themselves and interviewed all of the prospective fellows. Separate invasive and noninvasive training tracks were joined into a comprehensive three year program; additional advanced programs were available in the interventional, imaging, and electrophysiology Sections. At this time the Cardiology training program was the fourth largest in the country. The Interventional Registry was replaced with the PTCA Registry, supervised by Jan Howell as a part of the Clinical Trials Unit. The CAVEAT[3] and EPIC[5] trials were completed. The CAVEAT trial showed the nonsuperiority of atherectomy over balloon angioplasty in treating atherosclerotic lesions, and the EPIC trial showed the benefit of GIIb/IIIa inhibitors in high risk angioplasty. The ACUTE[6] study began (Assessment of Cardioversion Using TEE)—to assess left atrial thrombi/"smoke" (spontaneous echo contrast) in atrial fibrillation. Heupler became Chairman of Cath Lab Quality Control Committee.

Before coming to Cleveland, Topol had approached Robert Beekman, Chief of Pediatric Cardiology at Michigan to join him in Cleveland, but reluctant to leave Ann Arbor, he referred him to Larry Latson of Texas

Children's Hospital in Houston who came to the Clinic in January 1993, replacing Rick Sterba as head of Pediatric Cardiology.

Also in 1993 Brian Griffin, arrived from Dartmouth's Mary Hitchcock Hospital, Killian Robinson came from Adelaide Hospital in Dublin, Ireland, Michael Lauer came from the Lahey Clinic in Burlington, MA, Curtis Rimmerman, a Cleveland native, came from the Krannert Cardiology Institute at Indiana University, and Fred Shaw, who trained at Henry Ford Hospital and at the University of Minnesota—all joined Clinical Cardiology. [8] Pieter Vandervoort a Belgian native, came from Massachusetts General Hospital to join Cardiovascular Imaging.

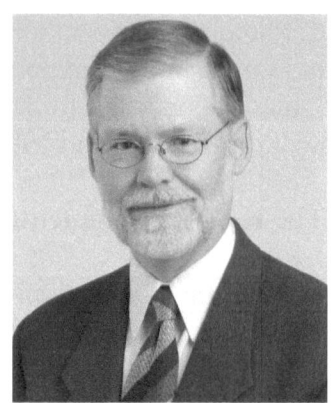

Larry A. Latson

To meet the needs of the internal medicine fellows assigned to Cardiology, the Ernstene and Shirey Teaching Services were established in 1993 under the Clinical Section. Staffing included rotating Staff cardiologists (largely from the Clinical Section) and a rotating Cardiology fellow. Further, two Surgical Services were created with several staff members, rotating from all sections, aided by clinical associate physicians, to cover surgical patients.

Tom Marwick, a native of Australia, had been a special Research Fellow in echocardiography since 1988, and had been was appointed to the staff in the Cardiac Function Lab in 1990. After a short hiatus to study in Europe he returned in 1993 to become Director of Stress Imaging.

The Joseph J. Jacobs Center for Thrombosis and Vascular Biology was established in 1993 in the Division of Research, with Topol as Chairman, and Edward Plow as its Director of Research. [9]

Griffin replaced Ian Black as Program Director in 1994. The number of fellow entering the program was increased to 14 per year, and the total complement of fellows was now 67 including advanced interventional, imaging and EPS fellows and Clinical and Research Fellows.

Michael Lincoff completed an interventional fellowship and joined the Interventional staff in 1994. [10] In college and medical school he had become interested in animal research. He continued his interest in animal studies, was one of the first to become interested in local drug delivery as a means of preventing restenosis and investigated a unique polymer coated stent in the animal lab.[7] Lincoff was named Director of the **Experimental Intervention Lab**. He developed many national and international contacts and soon became one of the Department's most prolific researchers.

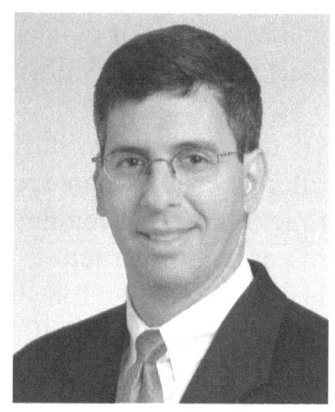

Michael Lincoff

New Staff members in 1994 included Pat Tchou, who came from the University of Pittsburgh to become Director of the Electrophysiology Laboratories, and subsequently Section Head when Lon Castle left for private practice in Elyria, Ohio. Tony DeFranco and David Moliterno joined the invasive Section upon completing Interventional Cardiology fellowships; Richard Grimm joined the Imaging Section after his fellowship in that subspecialty, and Mina Chung came from Barnes Hospital in St. Louis to join the EP section.

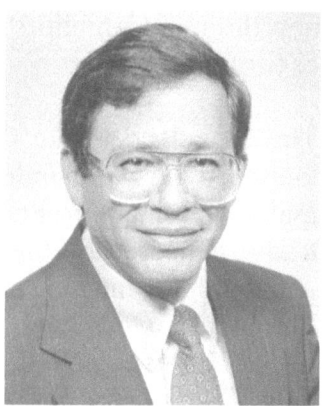

Patrick J. Tchou

Tchou created a section of basic research in cardiac electrophysiology in conjunction with molecular cardiology in the Research Division. This began with Igor Efimov who started as a Research Associate in 1994 and was appointed to the Assistant Staff in 1998 (ultimately departing for Case Western Reserve University in 2000 and later Washington University in St. Louis), Todor Mazgalev (1994) and David Van Wagoner(1996). Later additions to this group included Elena Sgarbossa (1995-1997), Yuan Na Cheng (1996), Donald Walick (1999), Mary Ruehr (2003) and Youhua Zhang (2003). This group made important contributions to the understanding of molecular changes related to cardiac arrhythmias and their response to defibrillation.

Of the many new staff members recruited by Topol with research interests, none had requested any officially sanctioned "protected time" that had been an issue in the previous administration. With the research infrastructure in place, Topol and colleagues became more involved with multicenter megatrials: GUSTO-I[2] continued, the first megatrial involving 40,000 patients with acute myocardial infarction (AMI) treated with either recombinant tissue plasminogen activator (r-TPA) or streptokinase; RESCUE-I[4], angioplasty after failed lytic therapy [11], CAVEAT-I[3], directional atherectomy versus angioplasty, GUSTO-II[8], angioplasty versus lytic therapy for AMI, and later EPIC[5], EPILOG[9] and EPISTENT[10], using abciximab (ReoPro) as an adjunct to interventional strategies, and still later REPLACE,[11] [12] a comparison of new thrombin inhibitors versus GIIb-IIIa antiplatelet agents (eptifibatide or tirofiban).

The Cleveland Clinic Cardiovascular Coordinating Center (C5) was launched in 1994 under the aegis of the Clinical Trials Unit as a multidisciplinary program to assist in coordinating multicenter clinical trials sponsored by the Clinic and other centers. The Clinic's ECG, Angiography, Imaging and IVUS core laboratories, the Homeostasis and Thrombosis Core Lab, and Biostatistics were key components of C5. In contrast to commercial research organizations, C5 coordinated trials only for academic institutions. It later became the coordinating center for all Cleveland Clinic trials.

Pediatric Cardiology Moves to Pediatrics

Doug Moodie had become Head of the Department of Pediatrics in 1986. Pediatric Cardiology remained a section in Cardiology until 1994 when it was transferred to the newly organized Division of Pediatrics, along with Larry Latson, Rick Sterba and Dan Murphy (The Cleveland Clinic Childrens Hospital had been designated in 1987). Pediatric catheterizations continued to be performed in the Cardiac Catheterization Laboratories, and Sterba, a pediatric electrophysiologist, continued to work also in the EP/Pacemaker Section.

Steve Nissen formalized an Intravascular Ultrasound Research Laboratory in 1994, and Murat Tuzcu had begun to do intracoronary ultrasound studies in post-cardiac-transplant patients in the cath lab.[12]

The Clinic had become the largest open-heart surgery center in the United States. In 1994 the 300th heart transplant was performed. The Department was featured on ABC's *Good Morning America* with the first live percutaneous intervention and intravascular ultrasound ever performed on network television.

In 1995 Dennis Sprecher arrived from the University of Cincinnati to head a new **Section of Preventive Cardiology**. Soon this section would include physicians from several departments: Mike Lauer, Fred Pashkow and Killian Robinson from Cardiology, Byron Hoogwerf (Endocrinology), Jeff Olin (Vascular Medicine), Don Vidt (Hypertension and Nephrology) and Cheryl Weinstein (Internal Medicine). The Cardiac Health Improvement and Rehabilitation Program (CHIRP) was transferred from the Imaging Section to the Preventive Cardiology Section in 1995 (later

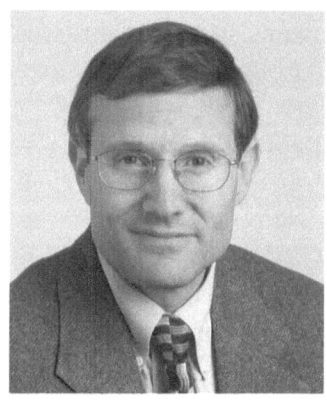

Dennis Sprecher

to be known as the Preventive Cardiology and Rehabilitation Section). Curt Rimmerman accepted an assignment as Director of the outreach program at Crown Center in Independence.

Topol had been looking for a nationally recognized leader in Heart Failure and Transplantation since he arrived. Jim Young was Director of the Heart Failure and Transplantation program at Methodist Hospital, Baylor University, in Houston, and well known for his research accomplishments. Topol called him on several occasions, and asked him for recommendations. Ultimately he convinced Young to visit Cleveland himself. Young knew Robert Hobbs who encouraged

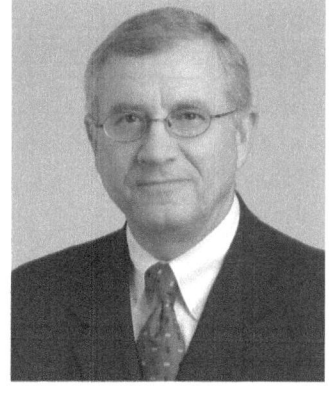

James B. Young

him to look at the program. Similarly impressed by what he saw at the Clinic, and with Topol's persuasiveness, Young agreed to become Head of the Section of Heart Failure and Transplantation, arriving in July 1995, succeeding Bob Hobbs. Young then recruited Randall Starling and Garrie Haas to join the Section, both coming from Ohio State University. He too organized his Section into rotating teams covering the outpatient clinic, hospital, and catheterization laboratory. One of his first projects was the development of an electronic medical record for heart failure patients that was integrated with a transplant registry. Another was to create a special fellowship in heart failure. Later a Heart Failure Intensive Care Unit was launched in the area formerly occupied by the coronary intensive care unit before the Century Project was completed.

Leonardo Rodriguez, who had been recruited by Thomas, joined the Imaging Section in 1995 after completing an advanced fellowship in that discipline. Mark Niebauer joined the EP Section having completed his Cardiology and EP fellowships at the University of Michigan. Also in 1995 an Atrial Fibrillation Clinic was initiated in the EP Section, directed by Mina Chung; Gregory Kidwell headed the EP Laboratory; Bruce Wilkoff headed the Implantable Device Clinic, and Vic Morant continued to head Arrhythmia Monitoring.

In 1995 cardiac surgeons began to perform minimally-invasive valve replacement procedures,[13,14] which proved particularly advantageous for isolated mitral valve replacements. Minimally-invasive and off-pump coronary artery bypass technics were explored. Surgical approaches for prevention and treatment of atrial fibrillation were also initiated.[15] By then Clinic surgeons were performing more valve operations each year than any other center in the US. The Imaging Section was identified as the lead center to coordinate digital acquisition and transmission of echocardiographic data aboard the International Space Station and began to work with NASA to develop echo algorithms to study the adaptation of the cardiovascular system to microgravity.

For the first time the US News and World Report ranked the Clinic No. 1 in the USA for Cardiology in 1995, and each year thereafter through 2006. [13]

Sorin Brener, a native of Romania and educated in Israel, completed his interventional fellowship and joined the Invasive staff in 1996. Richard

Trohman left to join the faculty of Rush University Medical Center in Chicago.

Mike Lauer succeeded Bruce Wilkoff as Director of the Cardiovascular Computing Unit. By this time the Cardiology Network included databases for all sections, patient files, support for nearly 500 staff, secretaries and other users, and a patient electronic medical record for the entire department was under development.

In 1997 Gary Francis came from the University of Minnesota to succeed Nissen as Director of the Coronary Intensive Care Unit (Mike Lauer became Associate Director). Suzanne Rodkey joined the Heart Failure Section. Sergio Pinski left for the Rush Medical Center in Chicago. [14] Mike Rollins and Sasan Ghaffari joined Clinical Cardiology (Ghaffari departed for California in 2004; Rollins currently works at the Independence facility). Loretta Isada and Ellen Mayer-Sabik joined the Imaging Section (Isada departed in 2003). Both were graduates of the cardiology training program and advanced imaging training programs. James Hodgman and William Sheldon both retired at the end of 1997.

All cardiology programs were asked to reduce their size because of an anticipated national oversupply in the future. The Clinic reduced the size of the first year program from 14 to 11 beginning in 1997. Ohio State medical students began rotating third year clerkships on the Ernstene and Shirey Teaching Services that continued under the supervision of Don Underwood.

The Kaufman Center for Heart Failure was established in 1997 to investigate the pathophysiology of heart failure and new treatments, with Jim Young as its Medical Director and Pat McCarthy, its Surgical Director.

After several years of development the electronic medical record was implemented in the outpatient clinics. The heart failure EMR was later integrated with the Cardiology-wide electronic medical record. Eugene Blackstone became Director of the Cardiovascular Information Registry (CVIR)

1998 brought five additions to the staff: Jay Yadav and Mitch Silver joined the Invasive/Interventional Section; Donald Hammer and Roger Mills joined the Clinical Section to oversee the two Surgical Services; and Joseph Frolkis joined Preventive Cardiology.

Yadav, trained first in neurology, came from the University of Alabama where he was trained in cardiology, and he also had expertise in carotid stenting; Mitch Silver was a graduate of the Interventional training program with added training in vascular interventions. He left for private practice in 2000. Ralph Augustini was a temporary Clinical Scholar in EP after completing an EP training program in 1998 but left after eight months and went to OSU. Tom Marwick returned to Australia in 1998, and where he has become a prolific researcher in cardiac imaging and stress testing as Professor of Medicine at the University of Queensland in Brisbane. Morant left on medical leave in May 1998 having sustained a debilitating cerebral hemorrhage. Fred Shaw left for Metro Health Center in December 1998. Darrell Dobowey also left in 1998.

The first phase of the Lerner Education and Research Building opened in 1998, fulfilling the vision of Bernadine Healy, nine years after the completion of the Sherwin Research Building in 1991. It would be completed in 1999 and provided, in addition to badly needed research space, new headquarters for the Education Division, the Medical Library, and new facilities for Biomedical Engineering.

In 1999 Andrea Natale and Walid Saliba joined the EP Section. Natale, a native of Italy, trained in Houston and London, Ontario, and was recruited from the University of Wisconsin. Saliba, from Lebanon, received cardiology training at Duke University and Baylor, and completed training in EP at the Clinic. Mohamed Yamani joined the HF Section in 1999 and Mathew Deedy joined the Clinical section; both were graduates of Cardiology programs.

Craig Asher had been a Clinical Associate in EP Research since 1997 after completing cardiology and imaging training; in 1999 he joined the staff in the Imaging Section. Fred Pashkow left in 1999 to become Medical Director of the Queens Medical Center Heart Institute in Honolulu, Hawaii, and Greg Kidwell left for private practice. Lon Castle returned, dividing his activities between the EP Section and at Lakewood Hospital through the Department of Regional Medicine.

Topol was beginning to look upon genetic medicine as a potentially exciting new area of investigation, and had launched a survey of over 400 families with premature coronary artery disease beginning in 1996. This became known as the GENEQUEST, a multicenter project. A genetic analysis of these individuals was performed in the laboratory of Quin Wang. A single-center GENEBANK project was initiated in 1998 to include 10,000 patients. A patient from Iowa was discovered with 21 immediate relatives who shared a common gene, MEF2A, which contained a deletion mutation, and seemed to be associated with premature heart attack.[16] The following year another gene mutation (thrombospondin-4 A387P polymorphism) was found that seemed to be a risk factor for coronary heart disease.[17] In the same year Topol, Edward Plow, David Moliterno and colleagues published results from Genequest,[18] that positioned Topol and his colleagues for a flagship NIH SCCOR grant of $18 million in 2004. Thus began a major thrust in genomic cardiology. Since then six more genes associated with premature heart attack have been identified. The effort continues with Stan Hazen, who joined Preventive Cardiology and is its current Head, as the Director of Genebank.

By 1999 Clinic electrophysiologists had accumulated one of the nation's largest experiences with internal cardioverter devices and were leaders in developing dual chamber pacemakers, and were key contributors to the AVID and DAVID trials.[19,20] Through the leadership of Bruce Wilkoff, the Clinic was one of the leading centers in the world for pacemaker lead extractions,[21] and bi-ventricular pacing program was initiated as an aid to the management of congestive heart failure.[22]

The EPISTENT trial was concluded and demonstrated the benefit of abciximab in patients undergoing PCI with stents.[23]

In research published in JAMA, Cleveland Clinic investigators led by Michael Lauer shed light on the implications of an abnormal cardiac response that occurs during exercise stress testing and nuclear imaging of the heart. They found that an impaired chronotropic response to exercise, and especially a slow heart rate recovery time after exercise, are important predictors of mortality in persons with known heart disease. Moreover, the combination of these abnormal heart rate responses and abnormal imaging results identified patients at high risk for coronary

William C. Sheldon, M.D.

events who should have aggressive management.[24,25] Young and his colleagues in the Heart Failure Section were involved in many local and multicenter clinical trials. Young served as Principal Investigator or Co-PI for many, including HOPE,[26] RESOLVED,[27] MIRACLE-ICD,[28] CHARM,[29] and OPTIMIZE-HF[30.] (also SCD-HeFT, ACCLAIM). Young was President of the International Society for Heart and Lung Transplantation in 2001.

In 1999 the Clinical Staff in the Department of Cardiology numbered 59. Ten years had elapsed since the completion of the Century Project in 1989, and fifteen years since completion of the major expansion in 1974. It was by now apparent that existing facilities would be inadequate to support continued growth of the Department and the Clinic began to plan for a new Cardiovascular Institute that would open in 2007-08.

After eight years Topol had become highly respected for his organizational skills, his research vision, and as a gifted teacher. His section heads had considerable freedom in directing their sections. He regularly met with the fellows and attended teaching conferences. He usually obtained most of the resources that he requested: Foundation support for personnel, facilities and equipment, and industry support for research. [15] He had no aspirations for leadership positions in national societies. As one colleague put it:

> When you spoke to him you always had his full attention. He never forgot anything and you had to be careful what you told him—he had a mind like a steel trap. He was incredibly smart and was inspiring. He actively encouraged his staff and fellows. He was somewhat of a maverick but he knew how to motivate people, and was inspiring.[31]

He also recalled:

> One day at a journal conference a fellow was discussing a paper on C-reactive protein and its value as an indicator of prognosis in coronary heart disease. The paper concluded that it was less valuable than other prognostic indicators. Topol objected, praising the benefits of CRP. The fellow suddenly climbed upon

a chair and exclaimed loudly that "now I am as tall as you and can talk as loud as you can but CRP has little value!" Topol was as surprised as everyone else and all laughed about the event.[31]

Another recalled:

> Topol was eager to read papers that his staff had prepared. If you slid a manuscript under his door at 5:00 pm, Topol would review it and have a carefully reviewed and edited copy back in your office the next morning at 8:00 am.[32]

The Pursuit of a New Medical School

But in 2000 Topol was growing restless. Having accomplished all that he had set out to do at the Clinic, he missed the academic environment. The Ohio State affiliation had its shortcomings. He began to look for new challenges elsewhere, and considered positions as Dean at Stanford University School of Medicine, and CEO and Dean at Ohio State University Medical School. Bernadine Healy learned that he had interviewed at Ohio State, and soon Loop called Topol to his office to discuss his future. Informing Loop of his frustration with the lack of a medical school, Loop determined that the academic affiliation should be reexamined, and that Topol should take the lead. A task force was formed to study the issue that included Paul DeCorletto, Guy Chisholm, George Stark, Rob Kay and Loop.

Topol was appointed Chief Academic Officer of the Clinic in December, 2000, bringing the Division of Research and the Division of Education under his purview, while he continued as Chairman of Cardiology and Director of the Jacobs Center for Thrombosis and Vascular Biology. The Clinic resolved to pursue its own medical school program.

Staff additions in 2000 included Chris Bajer, Invasive/Interventional; Marc Penn and Dennis Rupp, Invasive/Diagnostic; Maran Thamilarasan, Imaging; Robert Schweikert, EP/Pacing; Wael Jaber, and Joel Holland, Clinical. Jaber later became a member of the Imaging Section also in 2003. Rupp came from the University of Kansas and is currently located at the Willoughby facility; Jaber, who had completed a Clinic fellowship in cardiac imaging and entered private practice in New York the previous year, was recruited back to Cleveland, and Holland was in private practice in Cleveland and is now located in Beachwood. Garrie Haas departed for private practice at Riverside Methodist Hospital in Columbus, and later joined the faculty at Ohio State Medical Center.

In 2000 Curtis Rimmerman succeeded Nissen as Head of the Section of Clinical Cardiology. The following year the Gus P. Karos Chair in Clinical Cardiovascular Medicine was established with Rimmerman as its first holder.

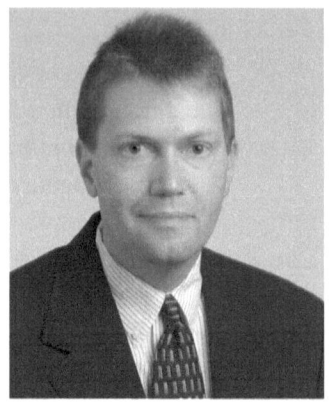

Curtis M. Rimmerman

In the Cath Lab the process was completed for converting from thirty-five millimeter cineangiographic films to digital acquisition and storage of cines. Motion picture films were no longer employed. The famous photographic reports that Sones had designed had been abandoned in the early 1990s and replaced with a computerized report. Also in 2000 Jim Young became the President of the International Society of Heart and Lung Transplantation.

New staff additions in 2001 included Depak Bhatt (Cath/Interv), David Martin (EP/Pacing), Raymond Migrino (Clinical/Heart Failure), David Taylor (Heart Failure), and Takahiro Shiota (Project Scientist in Imaging). Stan Hazen of Molecular Biology joined Preventive Cardiology (now known as the Section of Preventive Cardiology and Rehabilitation). Suzanne Rodkey left the Heart Failure Section for private practice.

In 2000 it had become apparent that the pulmonary veins could be the source of unusual electrical activity leading to atrial tachycardias. As this was explored further it was learned that these areas could be responsible for atrial fibrillation in many patients. Clinic electrophysiologists, led by Andrea Natale, were among the first to explore the feasibility of treating atrial fibrillation with radio frequency ablation of the pulmonary vein/left atrium interface.[33] By 2001 the EP section had become the fastest growing section in the Department with broadening application of automatic internal cardioverter/defibrillator devices, its landmark contributions in bi-ventricular pacing in the treatment of congestive heart failure, and pulmonary vein isolation for atrial fibrillation. Andrea Natale became

Co-Director of the Section of Electrophysiology and Pacing, with Pat Tchou.

Nissen was invited to join the Food and Drug Administration Advisory Committee on Cardiovascular Drugs in 2000. The first panel on which he participated, in February 2001, was to review Merck's anti-inflammatory drug Vioxx. Although the drug was approved, Nissen had reservations about the data. Debabrata Mukherjee, a cardiology fellow expressed interest and began to search FDA websites to study the data. In 2001, Mukherjee, Nissen and Topol published an analysis of the data that suggested an increased risk of cardiac complications with COX-2 inhibitors including Vioxx.[34] Topol became a vocal critic of Merck and the FDA. This had enormous ramifications leading to many legal actions against Merck. Topol was subpoenaed to testify in the first Federal case.

A fully configured echocardiograph was carried to the International Space Station, culminating a four year grant with NASA. Regrettably, two of the four astronauts who were trained to use the equipment were killed in the Columbia space shuttle disaster, and subsequent deferral of U.S. space missions left the space station with an acute shortage of manpower for conducting experiments on cardiac physiology.

Vascular Medicine Rejoins Cardiology

After forty-six years as a separate department, under Fay LeFevre, Victor DeWolfe, Jesse Young and Jeff Olin, successive chairmen, the decision

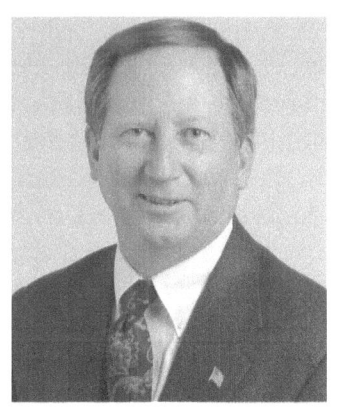

was made in 2001 to merge the Department of Peripheral Vascular Disease with Cardiology and the new department became known as the Department of Cardiovascular Medicine.

Thus Bill Ruschaupt, John Bartholomew, Susan Begelman, Carmen Fonseca, Lucy LaPerna and Felipe Navarro joined cardiologists Bajzer, Bhatt, Deichter and Yadav in a Section of Vascular Medicine, with Ruschaupt as Section Head. This came as a result of an unsuccessful search for a new Head of Peripheral Vascular Disease, and the vision of

William Ruschaupt

153

including both Vascular Medicine and Vascular Surgery in a Cardiovascular Institute as planning for the new building continued. Until then the Section and the Non-invasive Vascular Laboratory would remain at Desk S60 in the Main Clinic building. Peripheral interventions would continue in the catheterization laboratories. The training program in Vascular Medicine continued to be administered as a separate program in the Section of Vascular Medicine.

The Cleveland Clinic Lerner College of Medicine at Case Western Reserve University

During 2001 a number leaders from many distinguished academic institutions were invited to Cleveland to consult with the task force. Inasmuch as Ohio already had six medical schools [16] it seemed unlikely that a seventh would be approved by the Board of Regents or Ohio State Legislature, much less the ACGME, and any such effort would take years to accomplish. A medical school affiliated with CWRU might be more feasible. Loop, Topol, Malachai Mixon and Alfred Lerner met in Lerner's office with David Austin, then President of Case Western Reserve University, and members of the CWRU Board of Trustees. CWRU had been assessing its position. Although they had more then $200 million in NIH grants, they were far down on the list of academic institutions with NIH grants, which impaired their ability to attract top scientists. The Clinic had only about $70 million in NIH grants, but if this were to be combined with CWRU they would be near the top of the list. Austin and colleagues were interested in a possible affiliation. In the meanwhile Farah Walters and University Hospitals were interested in sharing the NIH grant credits with CWRU, and some of the CWRU Trustees were sympathetic to this, David Austin abruptly resigned as President. Lerner had been poised to make a major contribution to a conjoined medical school, but not without stable leadership at the University. It was not until Edward Hundert was named President of CWRU in May 2002 that Lerner was satisfied that a joint venture could succeed, and agreed to underwrite the project with a subsequent grant of $100 million. [17] The school was named the Cleveland Clinic Lerner College of Medicine of Case Western Reserve University and was dedicated to training physician scientists. Topol was Provost. A search committee, which included Topol, recommended the appointment of Ralph Horwitz of CWRU Dean in 2003, a year after the Medical College was created. The first class matriculated in 2004.

In 2002 Kenneth Shafer and Bennet Werner of the Wooster Clinic became members of the Clinical and Imaging sections four years after Wooster affiliated with the Cleveland Clinic in 1998.

Michael Rocco joined the Section on Preventive Cardiology in 2002 as Medical Director of Cardiac Rehabilitation and Stress Testing. Previously he had been at University Hospitals in Cleveland in a similar capacity.

Linda Graham joined the Section of Vascular Medicine and succeeded Bill Ruschaupt as Section Head. [18] Niebauer left EP for the University of Nebraska in 2002. Rupp left the Clinical Section for private practice. Migrino took a leave of absence in Clinical for an advanced fellowship in imaging at MGH, and subsequently accepted a position elsewhere.

Jim Young succeeded Nissen as Vice Chairman of Cardiology in 2002.

In the Interventional Section studies began on the use of beta- and gamma-radiation in the management of in-stent restenosis, and devices to prevent atheroemboli during carotid and vein graft interventions. The first drug eluting stents were employed (sirolimus and paclitaxol) in percutaneous coronary interventions. Per-catheter septal ablations were employed in the management of hypertrophic obstructive cardiomyopathy, and percutaneous closures of patent foramina ovalae and atrial septal defects were employed by pediatric cardiologists.

In 2003 Amjad AlMahameed Joined Vascular Medicine, and Lucy LaPerna departed. Stanley Hazen replaced Dennis Sprecher as Section head of Preventive Cardiology and Rehabilitation who left for the University of Pennsylvania. Cynthia Pordon and Paul Schoenhagen received joint appointments in the Clinical and Rehabilitation sections. Pordon graduated from the cardiology training program in 1990 (she worked in the Willoughby facility) and Schoenhagen completed a cardiology fellowship in 2002, followed by a year of CT/MR in Radiology. Caroline Casserly joined the Clinical Section in Westlake. Having completed interventional training at the Clinic in 2000 followed by a faculty appointment at the University of Washington and VA Hospital in Seattle, Samir Kapadia returned to the Invasive Section as an interventional cardiologist. Robert Mosteller came from Metro Health Center to join the EP Section at CCF-Westlake. Elizabeth Saarel, a Pediatric Cardiologist came from the University of Michigan to the Department of

Pediatrics with a joint appointment in the EP Section (but left a short time later). Nassir Marrouche joined the EP Section but also departed after a short time. Craig Asher left the Imaging Section for CCF Florida in 2003, and Loretta Isada left for private practice in Akron in 2003.

In November 2003 Jim Young became Chairman of the Division of Medicine, and was succeeded by Randall Starling as Head of the Heart Failure and Cardiac Transplant Section. (Young continued to see patients in that Section).

Also in November 2003, Nissen and colleagues published a the results of a small but important trial of recombinant apolipoprotein A-1 Milano that showed regression of coronary atherosclerosis in 47 patients with in acute coronary syndromes.[35] Three weeks later, at the AHA meeting he presented the initial results of the REVERSAL trial of aggressive LDL and CRP lowering through statin therapy.[36] These firmly established the Cleveland Clinic as a leader in the study of regression of coronary atherosclerosis.

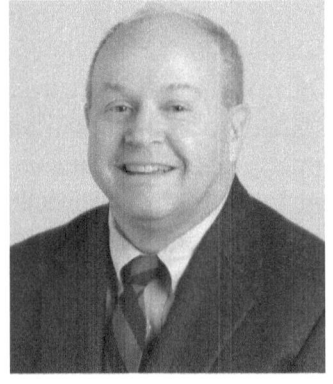

Gary Francis succeeded Rimmerman as Head of the Clinical Section in 2004. Eileen Hsich came from the Massachusetts General Hospital to join the Heart Failure Section in 2004. Wilson Tang received joint appointments in the Heart Failure and Invasive Sections having completed Cardiology and Heart Failure Fellowships in 2004.

Gary S. Francis

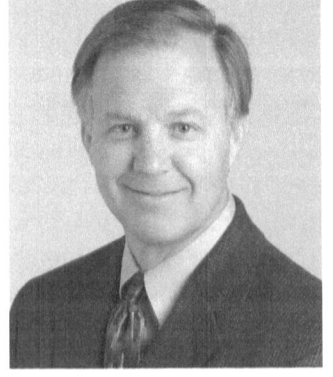

John Bartholomew

John Bartholomew succeeded Linda Graham as Head of the Section of Vascular Medicine. Completing a fellowship at Cleveland Clinic Florida, Teresa Carman joined that Section in 2004, as did Douglas Joseph after a Clinic fellowship in Vascular Medicine. Julie Huang joined Preventive Cardiology and Rehabilitation. Sreenivas Kamath joined the Invasive Section; Manuel Cerqueira was recruited from Georgetown University to become Head of Molecular and Functional Imaging in the Imaging Section. In 2004 the Department received a Specialized Center for Clinically Oriented Research (SCCOR) grant of $17.2 million over five years to study the role of genes and proteins in coronary artery disease. An additional $17 million was received from the founder of Medtronic for a new Brain-Heart program in conjunction with the Department of Neurosurgery.

The benefit of drug eluting stents was demonstrated in the TAXUS trial for which Steve Ellis was the principal investigator,[37] and Deepak Bhatt published a key paper in JAMA on the use of early invasive therapy in acute myocardial infarction (CRUSADE).[38]

Transition 1

Loop had attained age 65 in 2002, and by 2003 the planning of the Cardiovascular Research Institute building was well on it way, and in early 2004 he announced his intent to step down and retire. A search committee was formed consisting of trustees as well as members of the Board of Governors. There were seven candidates including Cosgrove and Topol.

From *To Act as a Unit*:[39]

> Finally, on June 2, 2004, Board of Trustees Chairman A. Malachi Mixon III announced the election of Delos M. "Toby" Cosgrove as the Clinic's next chief executive officer. Cosgrove had succeeded Loop as chairman of cardiovascular surgery, and would now succeed him again as CEO. This would be the Clinic's smoothest succession at the top leadership position, and the staff enthusiastically welcomed the transition.

> The combination of new divisional and departmental leadership as well as dynamic leadership at the top has kept the organization's energy level at high intensity. Coupled with the World Class Service leadership development initiative that began in 2003, these changes promise to catapult The Cleveland Clinic and the Cleveland Clinic Health System to new heights of accomplishment in the decades to come.

In 2005 Andrea Natale was named Director of the Electrophysiology Laboratories. Maurice Arruda, Mandeep Bhargava and Jennifer Cummings joined the EP section. Heather Gornick joined the Clinical/Vascular sections.

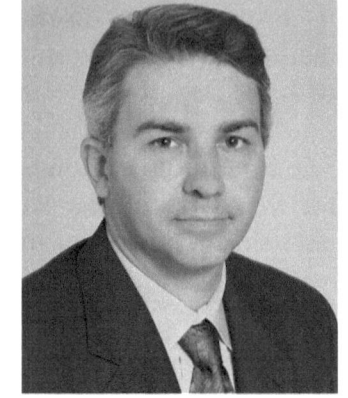

Andrea Natale

Leslie Cho had been a fellow in Cardiology and Interventional Cardiology graduating in 2002, after which she joined the faculty at Loyola University as Director of Carotid Interventions and Interventional Cardiology Research. In 2005 she returned to the Clinic to become Medical Director of Preventive Cardiology and the Women's Cardiovascular Center. She had a joint appointment in the Invasive/Intervention Section.

New additions to the Imaging Section in 2005 included Milind Desai, Chiara Leguori, Venuy Menon, and Srikanth Sola. Desai came from fellowships at Johns Hopkins and NIH. Legouri came from fellowships at the University of Pittsburgh (Heart Failure and Transplantation) and Columbia University (Advanced Echocardiography). Menon came from the University of North Carolina where he was Director of the Coronary Care Unit, and Director of the Chest Pain Clinic. Sola came from a cardiology fellowship at Emory University. Ajay Bhargava joined the Clinical Section after completing a fellowship at the University of Chicago, and Richard Krasuski arrived after his fellowship at Duke. Arman Askari, Vidyasagar Kalahasti and Timothy Williams joined the Clinical Section in 2005 after completing Clinic fellowships.

Transition 2

By 2004 the media and legal frenzy against Merck and Vioxx had reached a peak. Topol had become a consultant to an investment firm that had profited by short-selling shares of Merck based on information that he had collected and published three years previously. Although he denied any knowledge or participation in the fund's investments, and there was no evidence that he had profited from this position, conflict-of-interest accusations arose. He promptly resigned from this consultancy and all other industry ties.

In December 2005 the *Wall Street Journal* reported on Topol's testimony in the high profile case against Merck over Vioxx. Shortly after, in a reorganization to "streamline" Clinic administration Cosgrove eliminated the position of Chief Academic Officer and Provost of the medical school. As a result of this Topol lost his seat on the Board of Governors and other key committees and he quietly began looking for new opportunities elsewhere.

In February 2006, Topol resigned from the Staff of the Cleveland Clinic. He accepted an interim position as Professor of Genetics at Case Western Reserve University. Steve Nissen, who was then President Elect of the American College of Cardiology, was appointed Acting Chairman of the Department of Cardiovascular Disease, and a search committee was formed to find a new Chairman. On August 7, 2006 the Board of Governors announced that Nissen would be the new Chairman of Cardiovascular Medicine.

On October 23, 2006 the Scripps Institute, of San Diego California announced that Topol had accepted a position as Chief Academic Officer, Chief of Genomic Medicine and Translational Science Institute and Consultant in Cardiology, beginning January 1, 2007.

Thus ended fifteen years of major growth and accomplishment in Cardiology at the Cleveland Clinic. Topol proved to be an extremely bright, productive, and charismatic visionary. Topol's example in teaching, research and writing set a high mark for others to follow. During his tenure the Cardiology staff grew from 36 to 90, and the number of fellows grew from 45 to 66. Fifty of his fellows received prestigious faculty appointments at major universities and medical centers. The practice of cardiology was radically changed. Individual practices and referral patterns of the previous 59 years were deëmphasized in favor of institutional referrals. Clinical research increasingly played a key role for the Department, and basic research was now integrated; external funding for both became an important source of revenue. Whether patient satisfaction was preserved or improved is difficult to say, but patient activity and financial productivity continued to grow—not so much by increased individual productivity but by larger numbers of staff. The Department's technological innovations and research accomplishments were too massive to enumerate. In Topol's fifteen years he produced no fewer than 31 major books of cardiology including two textbooks in cardiovascular medicine and interventional cardiology, with subsequent updates, 147 book chapters, and co-sponsored the leading cardiology website, *theheart.org*. He contributed nearly 800 publications and 36 multicenter trial publications to peer reviewed literature.

He became a member of the Institute of Medicine of the National Academy of Science and the Association of American Physicians. And the Clinic's Cardiology program was consistently ranked No. 1 by the US News and World Report since 1995, with the strength of the Clinic environment and contributions from Cardiac Surgery.

During these fifteen years the face of American Medicine also changed. The transition of medical schools and centers from academic to corporate entities continued. Patient care revenues and NIH funding were no longer sufficient to support research and industry became more important than ever in supplementing these revenues, eclipsing support from the NIH. Megatrials became the *sine qua non* for establishing the role of new drugs and devices. The ethics of medical research was no longer to be taken for granted as researchers in academic and nonacademic medical centers sought professional and financial recognition. The "art" of medicine gave way to the "business" of medicine.

With the legacy of Eric Topol and the many vital staff members he left in Cardiology, The Cleveland Clinic had become irrevocably changed as it embarked upon the new venture of a Cardiovascular Institute.

Notes to The Topol Years

1. O'Neill had left to head the program at William Beaumont Hospital in Troy, Michigan.
2. Having established a liaison with Genentech in 1984 while a special fellow in coronary angioplasty at the San Francisco Heart Institute, Topol returned to Johns Hopkins, where he was the first to infuse TPA into a patient with acute myocardial infarction, [Collen D, Topol EJ, Tiefenbrunn AJ, Gold HK, Weisfeldt ML, Sobel BE, Leinbach RC, Brinker JA, Ludbrook PA, Yasuda T, Bulkley BH, Robinson AK, Hutter AM, Bell WR, Spadaro JJ, Khaw BA, Grossbard EB: Coronary thrombolysis with recombinant human tissue-type plasminogen activator: a prospective, randomized, placebo-controlled trial. Circulation 70: 1012-1017, 1984.]
3. Valentine Fuster, Chief of Cardiology at MGH warned Thomas that a move to Cleveland would ruin his career.
4. However Loop would not commit Clinic funds nor allow existing Cardiology funds to be used in support of a Cardiology Research Program, nor would he allow any portion of excess Cardiology clinical revenue to be directed toward the program. Funding had to be obtained externally.
5. One Cardiology staff member had met Topol in a men's room and despaired over the current state of affairs: "the sky (was) falling."
6. Healy was President of the American Heart Association in 1988-1999. She served as Director of the NIH until 1993 when she became Dean of the Ohio State University College of Medicine. A bid for the United States Senate in 1994 was unsuccessful. After a brush with a brain tumor she was named President of the American Red Cross in 1999, a post she held until 2001. Currently she is Health Editor for the U.S. News and World Report.
7. Some early recruitees will recall the super efficiency of Topol's first secretary, Jutta White, in making their travel arrangements, meeting them at the airport, and prompt reimbursement of expenses. Jutta also managed the arrangements for visiting professors and she served as his assistant when he traveled to meetings.
8. Shaw also headed the Consultation Service from 1995-1998.
9. By 1993 the organizational structure for the Department had been revised as follows:

Invasive Cardiology
   Steve Ellis, Section Head
   Sones Cardiac Catheterization Laboratories—Steve Ellis
   Interventional Cardiology—Pat Whitlow

Clinical Cardiology
   Steve Nissen, Section Head
   Coronary Intensive Care Unit—Steve Nissen
   ECG—Don Underwood
   Consultation Service—Fred Pashkow
   Ernstene and Shirey Teaching Services—Don Underwood
   Intravascular Ultrasound—Steve Nissen

Cardiovascular Imaging
   Jim Thomas, Section Head
   Echocardiography Laboratory—Bill Stewart, Director,
      Alan Klein—Associate Director
   Exercise Testing and Cardiac Rehabilitation—Fred
      Pashkow; Gordon Blackburn—Co-director of Cardiac
      Rehabilitation
   Imaging Research—Alan Klein
   Valve Management Center—Brian Griffin, Medical
      Director

Electrophysiology and Pacing
   Lon Castle, Section Head
   Holter Monitoring and Telemetry—Victor Morant

Heart Failure and Transplant Section
   Robert Hobbs, Section Head

Pediatric and Congenital Cardiology
   Larry Latson, Section Head

Experimental Interventional Laboratory—Mike Lincoff

Angiography Core Lab—Steve Ellis, Darrell Dobowey, Co-
directors

Center for Thrombosis and Vascular Biology—Eric Topol, Chairman, Edward Plow, Director of Research

Clinical Trials Unit—Sue Ann Deluca RN

Clinical Investigations (Grants Oversight) Unit—Val Stosik, MBA

Cardiology Graphics and Design—Darrel Debowey

Cardiovascular Computing Unit—Bruce Wilcoff

10. Lincoff recalls that his first case as an interventional fellow was with Pat Whitlow. While performing a catheter exchange he inadvertently dropped an expensive balloon catheter on the floor—and was devastated. To his credit, Whitlow said nothing, and simply requested another catheter, and the procedure continued uneventfully.
11. Ellis had started this study when he was at Michigan.
12. Lincoff was Principal Investigator of REPLACE.
13. This reflects not only Cardiology, but also the reputation of Cardiac Surgery and the entire Clinic environment—(many factors are considered in the *US News and World Report* rankings).
14. Pinski later returned to CCF Florida in 2002 as head of the section of Pacing and Electrophysiology.
15. Any snags in approval of requests for personnel or equipment were usually ascribed to the Division of Medicine office, although Dr. Muz Ahmad, Chairman of the Division, aways gave Topol *carte blanch.*
16. Extant medical schools were at Ohio State, Case Western Reserve, Cincinnati, Toledo, NEOUCOM, and Ohio U.
17. This was one of the largest contributions ever made to an academic medical institution in this country. Lerner was ill with a brain tumor at the time and died five months later on October 23, 2002.
18. Graham is a vascular surgeon who joined the Clinic Staff in 1999. She also holds appointments in Biomedical Engineering of the Lerner Research Institute.

References to The Topol Years

1. Topol EJ, Califf RM, Kereiakes DJ, George BS: Thrombolysis and Angioplasty in Myocardial Infarction (TAMI) trial. Journal of the American College of Cardiology. 1987;10:65B-74B.
2. Califf RM and Topol EJ for the GUSTO Investigators: Thrombolytic therapy for myocardial infarction: a perspective of clinical trialists. Clinical Cardiology. 1992;15:143-144.
3. Topol EJ, Leya F, Pinkerton CA, Whitlow PL, Hofling B, Simonton CA, Masden RR, Serruys PW, Leon MB, Williams DO, et al: A comparison of directional atherectomy with coronary angioplasty in patients with coronary artery disease. The CAVEAT Study Group. N Engl J Med. 1993;Jul 22;329(4):221-7.
4. Ellis SG, Ribeiro da Silva E, Heyndrickx G, Talley JD, Cernigliaro C, Steg G, Spaulding C, Nobuyoshi M, Erbel R, Vassanelli C, Topol EJ for the RESCUE Investigators: Randomized comparison of rescue angioplasty with conservative management of patients with early failure of thrombolysis for acute anterior myocardial infarction. Circulation. 1994;90:2280-2284.
5. The EPIC Investigators. Use of a monoclonal antibody directed against the platelet glycoprotein IIb/IIIa receptor in high-risk coronary angioplasty. The New England Journal of Medicine. 1994;330:956-961,
6. Klein AL, Grimm RA, Black IW, Leung DY, Chung MK, Vaughn SE, Murray RD, Miller DP, Arheart KL: Cardioversion guided by transesophageal echocardiography: The ACUTE pilot study. A randomized, controlled trial. Assessment of Cardioversion Using Transesophageal Echocardiography. Ann Intern Med. 1997; Feb 1;126(3):200-9.
7. Lincoff AM, Furst JG, Ellis SG, Topol EJ: Sustained local drug delivery by a novel intravascular eluting stent to prevent restenosis in the porcine coronary artery. JACC. 1994:18A. Poster presented at the American College of Cardiology Annual Scientific Sessions, 1994.
8. The GUSTO IIa Investigators: Randomized trial of intravenous heparin versus recombinant hirudin for acute coronary syndromes. Circulation. 1994;90:1631-37.
9. EPILOG Investigators: Effect of the platelet glycoprotein IIb/IIIa receptor inhibitor abciximab with lower. heparin dosages on ischemic complications of percutaneous coronary revascularization. New England Journal of Medicine. 1997;336:1689-96.
10. EPISTENT Investigators. Randomized placebo-controlled and balloon-angioplasty-controlled trial to assess safety of coronary stenting with use of platelet glycoprotein IIb/IIIa blockade. The Lancet. 352:87-92, 1998.

11. Lincoff AM, Topol EJ, for the REPLACE-2 Investigators: Glycoprotein IIb/IIIa inhibition in percutaneous coronary interventions. JAMA. 2003; 290:1451.

12. Tuzcu EM, De Franco AC, Hobbs R, Rincon G, Bott-Silverman C, McCarthy P, Stewart R, Nissen SE: Prevalence and distribution of transplant coronary artery disease: insights from intravascular ultrasound imaging. J Heart Lung Transplant. 1995;Nov-Dec;14(6 Pt 2):S202-7.

13. Cosgrove DM 3rd, Sabik JF: Minimally invasive approach for aortic valve operations. Ann Thorac Surg. 1996;Aug;62(2):596-7.

14. Navia JL, Cosgrove DM 3rd: Minimally invasive mitral valve operations. Ann Thorac Surg. 1996; Nov;62(5):1542-4.

15. McCarthy PM, Castle LW, Maloney JD, Trohman RG, Simmons TW, White RD, Klein AL, Cosgrove DM 3rd: Initial experience with the maze procedure for atrial fibrillation. J Thorac Cardiovasc Surg. 1993;Jun;105(6):1077-87.

16. Wang L, Fan C, Topol SE, Topol EJ, Wang Q: Mutation of MEF2A in an inherited disorder with features of coronary artery disease. Science. 2003;302:1578-81.

17. Narizhneva NV, Byers-Ward VJ, Quinn MJ, Zidar FJ, Plow EF, Topol EJ, Byzova TV: Molecular and functional differences induced in thrombospondin-1 by the single nucleotide polymorphism associated with the risk of premature, familial myocardial infarction. Journal of Biological Chemistry. 2004;279:21651-57.

18. McCarthy JJ, Parker A, Moliterno DJ, Salem R, Wang Q, Plow EF, Rao S, Shen G, Rogers WJ, Newby LK, Cannata R, Glatt K, Topol EJ, for the GENEQUEST Investigators: Large-scale association analysis for identification of genes underlying premature coronary heart disease: Cumulative perspective from analysis of 111 candidate genes. Journal of Medical Genetics. 2004; 41:334-41.

19. Kim SG, Hallstrom A, Love JC, Rosenberg Y Powell J, Roth J, Brodsky M, Moore R, Wilkoff B: Comparison of clinical characteristics and frequency of implantable defibrillator use between randomized patients in the Antiarrhythmics Vs Implantable Defibrillators (AVID) trial and nonrandomized registry patients. Am J Cardiol. 1997; 80(4):454-7.

20. Wilkoff BL: The Dual Chamber and VVI Implantable Defibrillator (DAVID) Trial: rationale, design, results, clinical implications and lessons for future trials. Card Electrophysiol Rev. 2003; (4):468-72.

21. Smith HJ, Fearnot NE, Byrd CL, Wilkoff BL, Love CJ, Sellers TD: Five-years experience with intravascular lead extraction. U.S. Lead Extraction Database. Pacing Clin Electrophysiol. 1994; Nov;17(11 Pt 2):2016-20.

22. Dresing TJ, Natale A: Congestive heart failure treatment: The pacing approach. Heart Failure Reviews. 2001;6(1):15-25.

23. *The* EPISTENT Investigators. Randomised placebo-controlled and balloon-angioplasty-controlled trial to assess safety of coronary stenting with use of platelet glycoprotein-IIb/IIIa blockade. The EPISTENT Investigators. Evaluation of Platelet IIb/IIIa Inhibitor for Stenting. Lancet. 1998; Jul 11;352(9122):87-92.

24. Lauer MS, Francis GS, Okin PM, Pashkow FJ, Snader CE, Marwick TH: Impaired chronotropic response to exercise stress testing as a predictor of mortality. JAMA. 1999;Feb 10;281(6):524-9.

25. Cole CR, Foody JM, Blackstone EH, Lauer MS: Heart rate recovery after submaximal exercise testing as a predictor of mortality in a cardiovascularly healthy cohort. Ann Intern Med. 2000:Apr 4;132(7):552-5.

26. The HOPE Study Investigators (Young JB: United States Study Co-Coordinator): Effects of an angiotensin converting enzyme inhibitor, ramipril, on death from cardiovascular causes, myocardial infarction, and stroke in high-risk patients. N Engl J Med. 2000;343:145-153.

27. McKelvie RS, Rouleau JL, White M, Afzal R, Young JB, Maggioni AP, Held P, Yusuf S: Comparative impact of enalapril, candesartan or metoprolol alone or in combination on ventricular remodelling in patients with congestive heart failure. Eur Heart J. 2003;Oct;24(19):1727-34.

28. Young JB, Abraham WT, Smith AL, Leon AR, Lieberman R, Wilkoff B, Canby RC, Schroeder JS, Liem LB, Hall S, Wheelan K; Multicenter InSync ICD Randomized Clinical Evaluation (MIRACLE ICD) Trial Investigators: Combined cardiac resynchronization and implantable cardioversion defibrillation in advanced chronic heart failure: the MIRACLE ICD Trial. JAMA. 2003;May 28;289(20):2685-94.

29. Young JB, Dunlap ME, Pfeffer MA, Probstfield JL, Cohen-Solal A, Dietz R, Granger CB, Hradec J, Kuch J, McKelvie RS, McMurray JJ, Michelson EL, Olofsson B, Ostergren J, Held P, Solomon SD, Yusuf S, Swedberg K; Candesartan in Heart failure Assessment of Reduction in Mortality and Morbidity (CHARM) Investigators and Committees: Mortality and morbidity reduction with Candesartan in patients with chronic heart failure and left ventricular systolic dysfunction: results of the CHARM low-left ventricular ejection fraction trials. Circulation. 2004;Oct 26;110(17):2618-26. Epub 2004 Oct 18.

30. Fonarow GC, Abraham WT, Albert NM, Stough WG, Gheorghiade M, Greenberg BH, O'Connor CM, Sun JL, Yancy C, Young JB; OPTIMIZE-HF Investigators and Coordinators: Carvedilol use at discharge in patients

hospitalized for heart failure is associated with improved survival: an analysis from Organized Program to Initiate Lifesaving Treatment in Hospitalized Patients with Heart Failure (OPTIMIZE-HF). Am Heart J. 2007;Jan;153(1):82. e1-11.

[31.] Griffin B. Personal communication 1/16/07.

[32.] Thomas J. Personal communication 3/13/07.

[33.] Natale A, Pisano E, Shewchik J, Bash D, Fanelli R, Potenza D, Santarelli P, Schweikert R, White R, Saliba W, Kanagaratnam L, Tchou P, Lesh M: First human experience with pulmonary vein isolation using a through-the-balloon circumferential ultrasound ablation system for recurrent atrial fibrillation. Circulation. 2000;102 (16):1879-82.

[34.] Mukherjee D, Nissen S, Topol EJ. Risk of cardiovascular events associated with selective COX-2 inhibitors: Journal of the American Medical Association, 2001;286:954-59.

[35.] Nissen SE, Tsunoda T, Tuzcu EM, Schoenhagen P, Cooper CJ, Yasin M, Eaton GM, Lauer MA, Sheldon WS, Grines CL, Halpern S, Crowe T, Blankenship JC, Kerensky R: Effect of recombinant ApoA-1 Milano on coronary atherosclerosis in patients with acute coronary syndromes: a randomized controlled trial. JAMA. 2003;290:2292-2300.

[36.] "REVERSAL," Late-Breaking Clinical Trials Plenary Session XI, American Heart Association Scientific Session, Orange County Convention Center, Orlando, Florida, November 12, 2003.

[37.] Stone GW, Ellis SG, Cox DA, Hermiller J, O'Shaughnessey C, Mann JT, Caputo R, Cohen DJ, Russell ME: The pivotal U.S. study of the slow-rate release polymer-based paclitaxel-eluting TAXUS stent in patients with De Novo coronary lesions: 1-year clinical results of the TAXUS-IV Trial. Circulation. 2003;108 (17): 533.

[38.] Bhatt DL, Roe MT, Peterson ED, Li Y, Chen AY, Harrington RA, Greenbaum AB, Berger PB, Cannon CP, Cohen DJ, Gibson CM, Saucedo JF, Kleiman NS, Hochman JS, Boden WE, Brindis RG, Peacock WF, Smith SC Jr, Pollack CV Jr, Gibler WB, Ohman EM; CRUSADE Investigators: Utilization of early invasive management strategies for high-risk patients with non-ST-segment elevation acute coronary syndromes: results from the CRUSADE Quality Improvement Initiative. JAMA. 2004;Nov 3;292(17):2096-104.

[39.] Clough JD, ed. *To act as a unit. The story of the Cleveland Clinic*. 4th ed. Cleveland: Cleveland Clinic Press; 2004.

EPILOG

During the seventy five years since Cardiology was inaugurated at the Cleveland Clinic, the practice of medicine in America has changed as never before. Forssman's self-catheterization of the right side of the heart occurred in 1929 while Ernstene was still a house officer in Boston. Before Ernstene's arrival in 1932 the Flexner Report of 1910 had already reduced the number of medical schools and proposed standards for admission and curricula. Medical specialties began to organize beginning in 1916. The seeds of "the Blues" medical and hospital insurance plans were sewn in 1917 and 1929 respectively. Small medical groups began to organize in the years after World War I. The Clinic was the second large multispecialty group to appear. Such groups were looked upon as threatening by private practitioners. Widespread organization of group practices did not occur until after World War II.

The American Boards of Medicine and Surgery were products of the mid 1930's. Specialties in medicine and surgery proliferated, especially in the years after World War II.

The Federal Government began to invest in medical research in the 1930's; NIH appropriations of $400,000 climbed to over $28 million in 1985. New drugs and technologies enhanced the practice of medicine and brought new sources of revenue, stimulating further investment but left many unable to cope with their added costs. The federal government entered the insurance field in 1965 with Medicare, and cost-plus reimbursement, feeding the medical economic engine with new revenue, new investment and building, and additional monies for research. This was a period of unparalleled growth, which could not be sustained.

Medicare reimbursement was revised according to disease-related groups (DRG's). Private insurers also revised their reimbursement formulas accordingly. New "managed care" entities emerged that were to rationalize reimbursement to physicians—PPO's, IPO's, and HMO's. None of these plans seemed to affect the growing number of uninsured individuals. Responding to a public demand government and private prescription drug plans were introduced that added to the costs.

During these years the practice of medicine—and cardiology—changed radically. Some scourge diseases began to decline if not virtually disappear: tuberculosis, with the advent of streptomycin and isoniazid; syphilis, rheumatic fever and rheumatic heart disease, with the introduction of penicillin; and poliomyelitis with the development of the Sabin and Salk polio vaccines (1953, 1955); smallpox had already been largely eradicated with the Jenner smallpox vaccine. Carcinoma of the stomach declined precipitously, with more effective management of peptic ulcer disease and other forces not clearly understood.

But new diseases were discovered—idiopathic hypertrophic subaortic stenosis (IHSS), mitral valve prolapse, coronary artery spasm, Alzheimer's disease, autism, and AIDS;—or resulted from new treatments: the post cardiotomy syndrome, post angioplasty restenosis, stent thrombosis, and cardiac transplant rejection.

In seventy five years The Cleveland Clinic became a major research center, and its Department of Cardiology has become one of the leading cardiovascular centers in the world. It is an amazing success story. The Clinic is recognized for many contributions of its Research Division to cardiovascular medicine including treatment of hypertension, hemodialysis and dietary management of hyperlipidemias. Clinic cardiologists introduced coronary arteriography, and made landmark contributions to the understanding the natural history of coronary artery disease. They have made important contributions to the technologies of cardiovascular imaging—angiographic, ultrasound, and radionuclear, and through their application, a better understanding of the diseases they serve. Cardiac electrophysiologists have advanced the management of cardiac arrhythmias and pioneered in cardiac pacemakers, defibrillators, automatic implantable cardiac defibrillators and ablation therapy for ventricular and atrial arrhythmias. Through large clinical trials Clinic cardiologists have expanded knowledge in technics of percutaneous coronary interventions, the understanding and prevention of post intervention restenosis, and pharmacological management of arrhythmias, heart failure, atherosclerosis, and the prevention of coronary disease.

Clinic surgeons are recognized for their contributions to open heart surgery—bypass graft surgery with vein and internal mammary (thoracic) artery technics, left ventricular assist devices and the implantable artificial heart programs, valve replacement surgery, valve repairs, heart and lung transplantation, and the study of ventricular remodeling for heart failure.

As the practice of cardiology has evolved from the individual practices of the first thirty years to a corporate/academic model in the past thirty years, patient relations have become somewhat less personalized, and staff relations less cohesive than in earlier years. Yet the Clinic is acknowledged for its team approach, productivity and unparalleled efficiency.

None of this could have been accomplished without the hundreds of staff physicians who worked long hours and sacrificed more lucrative careers they might have had in private practice. Cardiology's leaders—Ernstene, Proudfit, Sones, Sheldon and Topol, working with leaders in Cardiac Surgery—Effler, Loop, and Cosgrove have helped shape the vision, and set the direction, with the support of the Clinic's leaders—Crile, LeFevre, Wasmuth, Kiser, and Loop.

Now the Clinic is about to embark upon a new era with the creation of a new Cardiovascular Institute encompassing Cardiology, Cardiac Surgery, Cardiothoracic Anesthesiology, Vascular Medicine and Vascular Surgery, and their leaders. This will bring new challenges in maintaining efficiency in a larger organization, governance, communication, resource sharing and allocation, and responsible use of new technology while preserving the heritage of personalized patient care.

Inevitably there will be new challenges in the economics of health care as our government struggles with issues of rising costs, Medicare, the uninsured, increasing demand for research support, and tort reform. Fulfilling the curse of the ancient Chinese proverb: we live in interesting times!

But Cardiology and the Clinic have never been stronger, nor in a better position to deal with the uncertainties of the future, with its steadfast dedication to its mission to provide

> Better care of the sick
> Investigation of their problems
> Further education of those who serve.

APPENDIX 1

CARDIOLOGY STAFF PHYSICIANS

	From	To	Interest/Section
A C Ernstene, M.D.	1932	1967	Clinical/ECG
H S VanOrdstrand, M.D.	1939	1958	Pulmonary
Fay A. Levre, M.D.	1942	1955	Vascular
William L. Proudfit, M.D.	1946	1979	Clinical/ECG
David C. Humphrey, M.D.	1949	1959	Hypertension
John F. Whitman	1951	1960	Clinical/ECG
Richard N. Westcott, M.D.	1951	1973	Clinical/ECG
Victor G. DeWolfe, M.D.	1952	1955	Vascular
F. Mason Sones Jr., M.D.	1950	1983	Cath
Earl K. Shirey, M.D.	1957	1988	Cath
Royston C. Lewis, M.D.	1962	1992	Clinical/ECG
William C. Sheldon, M.D.	1963	1997	Cath
C. Charles Welch, M.D.	1965	1974	Clinical/ECG
David J.G. Fergusson, M.D.	1966	1969	Cath
James R Hodgman, M.D.	1966	1997	Clinical/ECG
Mehdi Razavi, M.D.	1967		Cath
Robert A. Quint, M.D.	1968	1971	Cath
Joel Webster, M.D.	1969	1973	Cath
John T. Huston, M.D.	1969	1972	Cath
Wayne Siegel, M.D.	1971	1977	Clin/CFL
Frederick A. Heupler, M.D.	1971		Cath
Y. Juan Lim, M.D.	1972	1992	Clin/ECG/CFL
Gustavo Rincon, M.D.	1972		Cath
Lon W. Castle, M.D.	1973, 1999	1994	Pace/EP
I.R. Rao, M.D.	1973	1975	Pace/EP
Augusto Pichard, M.D.	1973	1975	Cath
Charles Bost, M.D.	1973	1973	Cath
Hector Lardani, M.D.	1973	1977	Cath

Daniel F. Phillips. M.D.	1973	1983	Cath/Interv
Neil J. Hart, M.D.	1975	1982	Clinical/ECG
John R. Kramer, M.D.	1975	2002	Cath
Khosrow Dorosti, M.D	1975		Cath/Interv
Irving Franco, M.D.	1975		Cath/Interv
Ernesto E. Salcedo, M.D.	1975	1992	Clin/CFL
Victor Morant, M.D.	1976	1998	Pace/EP
Harry Lever, M.D.	1978		Clinical/ECG
Douglas S. Moodie, M.D.	1978	1995	PedCard
Robert E. Hobbs, M.D.	1979		Cath/HeartFail
Donald A. Underwood, M.D.	1980		Clinical/ECG
James D. Maloney, M.D.	1981	1992	Pace/EP
Conrad Simpfendorfer, M.D.	1982		Cath/Interv
Richard Sterba, M.D.	1982	1995	PedCard
Jay Hollman, M.D.	1983	1990	Cath/Interv
William J. Stewart, M.D.	1984		Clin/CFL
William A. Schiavone, D.O.	1984	1988	Clin/CFL
Gordon G. Blackburn, PhD	1985		Rehab
Bernadine Healy, M.D.	1985	1990	Research
Corrine E. Bott-Silverman, M.D.	1986		Cath/HeartFail.
Fuad Jubran, M.D.	1986		Clin/CICU
Philip J. Currie, M.D.	1986	1989	Clin/CFL
Tony Simmons, M.D.	1987	1992	Pace/EP
Patrick L Whitlow, M.D.	1987		Cath/Interv
Bruce Wilkoff, M.D.	1987		Pace/EP
Russell E Raymond, D.O.	1988		Cath/Interv
David VanWagoner, PhD	1988		EP Research
Paul Casale, M.D.	1989	1993	Cath/Interv
Richard Trohman, M.D.	1989	1996	Pace/EP
Frederick J. Pashkow, M.D.	1989	1999	Rehab

Name	Year	Year	Specialty
Allan L. Klein, M.D.	1990		Clin/Echo
Daniel J. Murphy, M.D.	1989	1995	PedCard
Fernando Grigera, M.D.	1990	1992	Cath/Interv
Thomas Marwick, M.D.	1990	1998	Clin/CFL
Eric J. Topol, M.D.	1991	2006	Cath/Interv
Stephen G. Ellis, M.D.	1991		Cath/Interv
Karen B. James, M.D.	1991		Heart Failure
Carol Duffy, M.D.	1992	1993	Imaging
Fetnat Fouad-Tarazi, M.D.	(1979 1992		Research) EP
James D Thomas, M.D.	1992		Imaging
Steven E Nissen, M.D.	1992		Clinical/CICU
E. Murat Tuzcu, M.D.	1992		Cath/Interv
Tom Karson, M.D.	1992	1994	Clinical
Joseph M. Sutton M.D.,	1992	1996	Cath/Interv
Ian Black M.D.,	1992	1994	Imaging
Gregory A. Kidwell, M.D.	1992	1998	Pace/EP
Brian Griffin, M.D.	1993		Imaging
Fredrick J. Jaeger Jr, D.O.	1993		Clinical/EP
Larry A. Latson, M.D.	1993	1995	PedCard
Killian C. Robinson, M.D.	1993	2000	Clinical
A. Michael Lincoff, M.D.	1993		Cath/Interv
Michael S. Lauer, M.D.	1993	2007	Clinical
Curtis M. Rimmerman, M.D.	1993		Clinical
Sergio L Pinski, M.D.	1993 2002	1995	Pace/EP Pace/EP/Florida
Pieter Vandervoort, M.D.	1993	1996	Imaging
W. Fred Shaw, M.D.	1993	1998	Clinical
Mina Chung, M.D.	1994		Pace/EP
Patrick J. Tchou, M.D.	1994		Pace/EP
Richard A. Grimm, M.D.	1994		Imaging
Anthony C. DeFranco, M.D.	1994	1996	Cath/Interv
David J. Moliterno, M.D.	1994	2003	Cath/Interv
James B. Young, M.D.	1995		HeartFailure
Randall Starling, M.D.	1995		HeartFailure
Mark J. Niebauer, M.D.	1995	2002	Pace/EP
Dennis L. Sprecher, M.D.	1995	2003	Preventive
Garrie J. Haas, M.D.	1995	2000	HeartFailure
Leonardo Rodriguez, M.D.	1995		Imaging
Sorin Brener, M.D.	1996		Cath/Interv
Mario J. Garcia, M.D.	1997	2006	Clin/Echo
Suzanne Rodkey Lutton M.D.	1997	2001	HeartFaillure

Name	Year	Year	Specialty
Ellen Mayer Sabik, M.D.	1997		Imaging
Sasan Ghaffari, M.D.	1997	2004	Clinical/Cath
Sergio Pinsky, M.D.	1997	1997	Pace/EP
Loretta Isada, M.D.	1997	2003	Imaging
Mark Kreindell, M.D.	1997		Cath
Gary Francis, M.D.	1997		Clinical/CICU
Mike Rollins, M.D.	1997		Clin/Imaging/ Independence
Stanley Hazen Ph.D.	1997		Preventive
Donald Hammer, M.D.	1998		Clinical/ Post op Surg
Jay S. Yadav, M.D.	1998	2006	Cath/Interv
Mitch Silver, M.D.	1998	2000	Cath/Interv
Joseph Frolkis, M.D. Ph.D.	1998	2001	Preventive
Roger M. Mills, M.D.	1998	2004	Clinical
Craig Asher. M.D. Florida	1999 2004	2003	Imaging
Mathew Deedy M.D.	1999	2004	Clinical/Cath
Andrea Natale, M.D.	1999	2007	Pace/EP
Walid Saliba, M.D.	1999	2008	Pace/EP
Mohamad Yamani, M.D.	1999		Heart Failure/Cath
Chriastopher Bajzer, M.D.	2000		Cath/Interv/Vasc
Joel Holland, M.D.	2000		Clin/Beachwood
Robert Schweikert, M.D.	2000	2008	EP
Wael Jaber, M.D.	2000 2003		Clinical Imaging
Mark S. Penn, M.D. PhD	2000		Cath/Clinical
Dennis Rupp, M.D.	2000		Cath/Clinical/ Prevent/ (Strongsville)
Maran Thamilarasan, M.D.	2000		Imaging
John Bartholomew, M.D.	(1998) 2001		Vascular Medicine
Susan Begelman, M.D.	(2000) 2001	2006	Vascular Medicine
Steven Deitcher, M.D.	(1998) 2001	2004	Vascular Medicine
Carmen Fonseca, M.D.	(1994) 2001	2004	Vascular Medicine
Lucy LaPerna, D.O.	(1997) 2001	2003	Vascular Medicine
Felipe Navarro, M.D.	2001	2002	Vascular Medicine
William Ruschaupt, M.D.	(1978) 2001		Vascular Medicine
Deepak L. Bhatt, M.D.	2001		Cath/Interv
David Martin, M.D.	2001		Pace/EP

Raymond Q. Migrino, M.D.	2001	2002	Clinical.
Takahiro Shiota, M.D.	2001		Imaging
David O. Taylor, M.D.	2001		Heart Failure
Michael Maier, D.P.M.	(2000) 2002		Vascular Medicine
Linda Graham. M.D.	(1999) 2002	2004	Vascular Medicine
Michael B. Rocco M.D.	2002		Clinical/Prevent/ Beachwood.
Dennis Rupp, M.D.	2002 2006	2004	Invasive Willoughby
Kenneth Shafer, M.D.	2002		Clinical/ (Wooster)
Bennett Werner, M.D.	2002		Clinical/ (Wooster)
Amjad AlMahameed, M.D.	2003	2006	Vascular Medicine
Caroline Casserly, M.D.	2003		Clinical/ (Westlake)
Stanley Hazen, M.D. PhD	(1997) 2003		Preventive
Samir Kapadia, M.D.	2003		Inv/Interv
Christine Moravec, PhD.	1993		Heart Failure Research
Robert Mosteller, M.D.	2003		EP/(Westlake)
Cynthia Pordon, M.D.	2003	2006	Clinical/Rehab/ (Willoughby)
John Burkhardt, M.D.	2004		EP
Teresa Carman, M.D.	2004		Vascular Medicine
Julie Huang, M.D.	2004		Clin/Preventive
Manuel Cerqueira M.D.	2004		Imaging
Eileen Hsich, M.D.	2004		Heart Failure
Sreenivas Kamath, M.D.	2004	2006	Clinical/Cath
Elizabeth Saarel, M.D.	2004	2005	EP/Peds
Mustapha Shaaraoui, M.D.	2004		Clin/Hospitalist
Wilson Tang, M.D.	2004		Heart Failure/Cath
Raghavendra Allareddy, M.D	2005	2008	Clin/Hospitalist
Mauricio Arruda, M.D.	2005	2007	EP
Arman Askari, M.D.	2005		Clinical
Mandeep Bhargava, M.D.	2005		EP
Ajay Bhargava, M.D.	2005		Clinical
Leslie Cho, M.D.	2005		Preventive/Interv
Jennifer Cummings, M.D.	2005		EP
Milind Desai, M.D.	2005		Imaging/CT&MR
Michael Faulx, M.D.	2005		Clinical
Heather Gornik, M.D.	2005		Clinical/Vascular

Vidyasagar Kalahasti, M.D.	2005		Clinical/ Post-op Surg
Richard Krasuski, M.D.	2005		Clinical
Chiara Liguori, M.D.	2005		Imaging
Thomas Lutz, M.D.	2005		Clin/Hospitalist
Venugopal Menon, M.D.	2005		Imaging/CICU
Girish Mood, M.D.	2005		Clin/Hospitalist
Derek Smith, M.D.	2005		Clin/Hospitalist
Srikanth Sola, M.D.	2005		Imaging/CT&MR
Timothy Williams, M.D.	2005	2007	Clinical
Terrence Tulisiak, M.D.	2005		Clinical/ (Strongsville)
Ashoka Nautiyal, M.D.	2005		Clin/Interv (Westlake)
Firas Al Solaiman, M.D.	2006		Vascular
Michael Maier, DPM	2000		Vascular
Douglas Joseph, D.O.	2004		Vascular
Venu Menon, M.D.	2005		Imaging
Mauricio Arruda, M.D.	2005	2008	EP
Thomas Dresing, M.D.	2006		EP
Oussama Wazni, M.D.	2006		EP
Thomas Edel, M.D.	2006		EP (Westlake)
Adriana Fodor, M.D.	2006		Clin/Hospitalist
Mazen Hanna, M.D.	2006		Heart Failure

*(List does not include Ph.D. researchers)

Cath = diagnostic cardiac catheterization
CFL = cardiac function laboratory (later Imaging)
CICU = coronary intensive care unit
Clinical = clinical cardiology
CT&MR = computerized tomographic and magnetic resonance cardiac imaging
ECG = electrocardiography
Heart Fail= heart failure
Interv = interventional cardiology
Pace/EP = pacemakers and electrophysiology
PedCard = pediatric cardiology
Post-op Surgical = postoperative surgical service
Pulmonary = pulmonary diseases
Rehab = cardiac rehabilitation

Vascular = peripheral vascular disease

APPENDIX 2

CARDIOLOGY FELLOWS, PROGRAM,
DATE OF COMPLETION

Kinell, Jack, MD	IM (Card)	1941
Proudfit, William Lyie, MD	IM (Card)	1943
Hofsteter, Grace, MD	Cath	1954
Hearn, Charles J., MD	ClinCard	1956
Shirey, Earl K., MD	Cath	1957
Cumming, Gordon, MD	ClinCard	1958
Garcia, Hector L., MD	ClinCard	1958
La Camera, Frank, Jr., MD	Cath	1959
Tapia, Fernando, MD	Cath	1959
Georgopoulos, Athan J., MD	ClinCard	1960
Kemp, V. Eric, MD	ClinCard	1960
Vlasteris, Philip A., MD	Clincard	1960
Lapointe, Leonard J. A., MD	Cath	1961
Sosa, Julio A., MD	Cath	1961
Lewis, Royston, MD FRCP	ClinCard	1962
Arnn, Edward, MD	ClinCard	1962
Baird, Charles L, Jr., MD	Cath	1962
Brewer, Timothy F., Ill, MD	Cath	1962
Sheldon, William C., MD	Cath	1962
Gould, David H., MD	Cath	1963
Hermann, Hector J. MD	Cath	1963
Kong, Thomas Q. MD	Cath	1963
Begg, Frank R., MD	Cath	1964
Demany, Martial, A. MD	Cath	1964
Franklin, Marshall, MD	Cath	1964
Michaud, Andre J. MD	Cath	1964
Macleod, Cathel A. MD	Cath	1959, 1965

Noto, Thomas J.,Jr.,MD	Cath	1965
Pritehard, George E., MD	Cath	1965
Tobon, Francisco, MD	Cath	1965
Fierens, Enrique, MD	Cath	1966
Gracey, JackG., MD	Cath	1966
Gulde, Robert E., MD	Cath	1966
Hodgman, James, MD	ClinCard	1966
Laman, Muryl L., MD	ClinCard	1966
Miller, Anthony, MD	Cath	1966
Miller, Giles, MD	Cath	1966
Scanlon, Patrick J., MD	Cath	1966
Schwid. Steven A. MD	ClinCard	1966
Stasis, Mohamed A.MD	Cath	1967
Azadeh, Houshang, MD	Cath	1967
Biagioni, Eugene, M., MD	Cath	1967
Cochran, Bertram H., MD	ClinCard	1967
Fiedotin, Arnoldo, MD	Cath	1967
Johnson, Charles D., MD	Cath	1967
Razavi, Mehdi, MD	Cath	1967
Siegel, Wayne, MD	ClinCard	1967
Cavanaugh, Richard K. MD	Cath	1968
Eipper, Donald F., MD	ClinCard	1968
Lequizamon, Enrique, MD	Cath	1968
Lim, Yee Juan, MD	ClinCard	1968
Quint, Robert, MD	Cath	1968
VanDenBroek, Hans, MD	Cath	1968
Bavikatty. Ramachandra, MD	Cath	1969
Borgese, Anthony C., MD	Cath	1969

Name	Type	Year
Grinfeld, Lillian, MD	ClinCard	1969
Huston, John T, MD	Cath	1969
Kolletis, Miltiades, MD	Cath	1969
Mathew, George M, MD	ClinCard	1969
Oddson, Gudmundur, MD	Cath	1969
Sayegh, Said, MD	Cath	1969
Abdelazim, Mohamad I., MD	Cath	1970
Hanna, Michael A., MD	Cath	1970
Jameson, Simon, MD	ClinCard	1970
Nourani, Dan K., MD	Cath	1970
Piessens, Jan H., MD	Cath	1970
Simpson, Carroll S., MD	Cath	1970
Stan, George, MD	Cath	1965, 1970
Swaye, Paul S., MD	Cath	1970
Aramburu, Socrates B., MD	Cath	1971
Creus, Antonio B, MD	ClinCard	1971
Dhanda, Satish K. MD	Cath	1971
DonMichael, T. Anthony, MD	Cath	1971
Germanovich, Ell, MD	Cath	1971
Hart, Neil J., MD	ClinCard	1971
Heupler, Frederick A., Jr., MD	Cath	1971
Khooblall, Khem L., MD,	ClinCard	1971
Leguizamon, Mario C., MD	ClinCard	1971
Miller, Roger D., MD	Cath	1971
Sequeira, Carmelindo Jr., MD.	Cath	1971
Seshagiri, Tippur N., MD	Cath	1971
Arakaki, Felix, MD	ClinCard	1972
Bost, Charles, MD	Cath	1972
Bruschke, Albert V.G. MD	ClinCard	1972
Durbeck, Donald C., MD	Cath	1972
Hajra, Bhrigu, MD	ClinCard	1972
Hardy, Geraldine, M., MD	ClinCard	1972
Kozul, Vlado, MD	Cath	1972
Lee, K.D., MD	Cath	1972
Moberg, Carl, H., MD	Cath	1972
Rincon, Gustavo, MD	Cath	1972
Shinji, Kumitsu, MD	Cath	1972
Yamaguchi, Hiroshe	Cath	1972
Berezovsky, Leonardo, A. MD	Cath	1973
Caplivski, Abraham, MD	Cath	1973
Castle, Lon W., MD	ClinCard	1973

Name	Type	Year
De La Rosa, Oscar, L. MD	Cath	1973
Kim, KyungSoo, MD	Cath	1973
Kramer, John Robert, Jr., MD	Cath	1973
Lardani, Hector, MD	Cath	1973
Philips, Daniel, MD	Cath	1973
Pichard. Augusto, MD	Cath	1973
Rao, Innanje Ravi, MD	Cath	1973
Rentrop, Klaus Peter, MD	Cath	1973
Rubenstein, Hector, MD	ClinCard	1973
Abe, Hiroyuki, MD	Cath	1974
Althouse, Bruce	Cath	1974
Betts, Duane, D., MD	Cath	1974
Dhawer, VIrender P.S., MO	Cath	1974
Dorosti, Khosrow, MD	Cath	1974
Fontenot, Joseph L, MD	Cath	1974
Franco, Irving, MD	Cath	1974
Gaal, Geza Z, MD	ClinCard	1974
Ishimori, Tetsuo, MD	Cath	1974
Kherani, Razak U., MD	Cath	1974
Lasko, Keith, MD	ClinCard	1974
Sthienchoak, Punnee, MD	Cath	1974
Andres-Pelaez, Leticia	Noninv	1975
Atassi, Keith, MD,	Inv	1975
Davies. Alien David, DO	Inv	1975
Duarte, Enio, MD	Inv	1975
Eikens, Eduards, MD	Inv	1975
El-Attar, Osamah A., PhD MD	Noninv	1975
Garvey, John MD	Inv	1975
Goyle, Krishan K., MD	Inv	1975
Kawamura, Kenzo, MD	Noninv	1975
Lamp, Lloyd M. MD	Noninv	1975
Lewis, John Randolph, MD	Inv	1975
Martin, Luis, MD	Inv	1975
Morcerf, Fernando, MD	Noninv	1975
Moreyra, Abel E., MD	Cath	1975
Petno, Vinceni, MD	Noninv	1975
Salcedo, Ernesto E., MD	Noninv	1975
Salgado, Carios A., MD,	Inv	1975
Shahamatpour, Ahmad, MD	Inv	1975
Tahmooressi, Parviz, MD	Inv	1975

Wojnar, Victor S. MD	Inv	1975	Kabel, David W., MD	Noninv	1978
Zureikat, Harran, M.D,	Inv	1975	Koizumi, Bradley H., MD	Noninv	1978
Abedin, Zainul, MD	Inv	1976	Kothari, Anil G., MD	Inv	1978
Arunthari, Cheerasak, MD	Inv	1976	Moghbeli, Homayoon G., MD	Inv	1978
Chalam, Venkata, MD	Inv	1976	Monteverde, John P, MD	Inv	1978
Fabre, Carlos, MD	NonInv	1976	Moon, Chae Hyun, MD	Inc	1978
Manubens, Sergio MD	Inv	1976	Persand, Eduardo, MD	Inv	1978
Morant, Victor, MD	Noninv	1976	Sakhaii, Mohsen, MD,	Inv	1978
Premsingh, Nalini, MD	Inv	1976	Salka, Mohamad G., MD	Inv	1978
Pumarino, Rene, MD	Inv	1976	Schareghi, Khosrow, MD	Inv	1978
Quiroga, Gary T, MD	Inv	1976	Seco, Jose E., MD	Inv	1978
Reddy, Amarenda, MD	Inv	1976	Sperber, Silvio B., MD	Inv	1978
Serrano-Munoz, Jose, MD	Inv	1976	Stiff, Dr. Philip C., Jr.	Inv	1978
Setty, Ramachandra, MD	Inv	1976	Tabbaa, Rashed, MD	Inv	1978
Singh, Kunwarjit, MD	Inv	1976	Thongouthaithip, Viyada, MD	Inv	1978
Siqueira, Dr. Carmelindo, Jr.	Noninv	1976	Uy,SantosA.,Jr.,MD	Inv	1978
Soares, Jocelino, MD	Inv	1976	Wattoo, Dost M.,MD	Inv	1978
Villamil, Ramon J., MD	Inv	1976	Yun, Joe H.,MD	Inv	1978
Wall, Rod, MD	Noninv	1976	Aronow, Martin R., DO	Inv	1979
Zachariah, Zachariah, MD	Inv	1976	Campbell, William B., MD	Inv	1979
Alavi, Mosen, MD,	Noninv	1977	Cramer, Charles W. MD	Inv	1979
Al-Hakim, Osama, MD	Inv	1977	Fredericka, David N, MD	Noninv	1979
Belardi, Jorge Atilio, MD	Inv	1977	Greer, Lowell, III, DO	Inv	1979
Bianchi, Federico, MD	Inv	1977	Gupta, Bhagwan D., MD	Inv	1979
Castor, Conrado P., MD	Inv	1977	Hashway, Thomas N. MD	Noninv	1979
Flores, Arturo	Noninv	1977	Henderson, Ray L., MD	Noninv	1979
Izquierdo, Pasqual, MD	Inv	1977	Herrada, Paul J, MD,	Inv	1979
Jonsson, Asgier, MD	Inv	1977	Hobbs, Robert E, MD	Inv	1979
Koo, Hugo, MD	Inv	1977	Mistry, Vijay Govindkant, MD	Inv	1979
Matsuda. Yasuo, MD	Inv	1977	Mulligan, John C., DO	Inv	1979
Motekallem, Mohammed, MD	Inv	1977	Pierce, Stephen A, MD,	Inv	1979
Shoukfeh, Mohammed F., M D	Inv	1977	Rao, Madhava S., MD	Inv	1979
Swami. T.C. Lakshmi, MD	Inv	1977	Razavi, Ali Seid, MD	Inv	1979
Warman, Vikram K., MD	Inv	1977	Ribic, John R., DO	Inv	1979
Zeni, Abdel, MD	Inv	1977	Simpfendorfer, Conrad C.,MD	Inv	1979
Alosilla, Carlos E., MD	Inv	1978	Sroujieh, Khaldoun S, MD	Inv	1979
Arditti, Jacques, MD	Inv	1978	Tansiongco, Ermel T, MD	Inv	1979
Boghairi, Anoush, MD	Noninv	1978	Dieterich, David D., DO	Inv	1980
DosSantos, Edgardo	Inv	1978	Hull, William L, DO	Inv	1980
El Tabbaa, Mohammad R. MD	Inv	1978	Lynch, James D., MD	Inv	1980
Japra, Romesh Kumar, MD	Inv	1978	McWilliams, Gregory J., DO	Inv	1980

Mellino, Marcelo M., MD	Inv	1980		Adams, Kenneth V. MD	Inv	1983
Millit, H. David, MD	Inv	1980		Chhabra, Anil, MD	Inv	1983
Nautiyal, Ashoka, MD	Inv	1980		Dorfman, Philip M, MD	Inv	1983
Quinn, James A, MD	Inv	1980		Duber, Roger, DO	Inv	1983
Raghavan, Prakash V. MD	Inv	1980		Eastway, Robert J., DO	Inv	1983
Rich, Stanley D. MD	Inv	1980		Kitazume, Hidemasa, MD	Inv	1983
Sebold, Ronald (Ron) C., DO	Inv	1980		Ng, Amy, MD	Inv	1983
Siegel, Marvin D. DO	Inv	1980		Raju, Namburu V. R., MD	Inv	1983
Underwood, Donald A. MD	Noninv	1980		Schiavone, William A. DO	Inv	1983
VanDenToren, Enoch W.,MD	Noninv	1980		Tsai, A. Roger MD	Inv	1983
Young. Stephen Paul, DO	Inv	1980		Abi-Mansur, Pierre S., MD	Inv	1984
Awan, Ihsan H., MD	Noninv	1981		Baker. Joseph C., MD	Noninv	1984
Awan, Ihsanul, A., MD	Noninv	1981		Corbelli, John C., MD	Inv	1984
Besley, Dennis C., MD	Inv	1981		Detrano, Robert C. MD	Noninv	1984
Brahmbhatt, Ramesh J., MD	Inv	1981		Gabis, Joseph MD	Noninv	1984
Ceimo, Joanne Mary, MD	Inv	1981		Haque, Ihsan Ul, MD	Inv	1984
ElTobgy, Sherif M.K., MD	Inv	1981		King-Rankine, Marilyn, MD	Noninv	1984
Modlinger, Ronald E., MD	Noninv	1981		Rollins, Michael B, MD	Noninv	1984
Pattison, R. Keith, DO	Inv	1981		Baum, Joan E. DO	Inv	1985
Primiano, Charles A., MD	Inv	1981		Beaver, Barney, B. DO	Inv	1985
Rao, Anantha K., MD,	Inv	1981		Bott-Silverman, Corinne, MD	Inv	1985
Schrader, Daniel D., MD	Noninv	1981		Ellis, John Henry, IV, MD	Inv	1985
Schwarz, Eugene F., MD	Inv	1981		Fisher, Russell G. DO	Inv	1985
Spears, James R., MD	Inv	1981		Fontaine, John M., MD	Inv	1985
Tegtmeier, Terry Emil, MD	Inv	1981		Haggman, Dale L. DO	Inv	1985
Walden, Emerson C., Jr., MD	Noninv	1981		Keyser, Philip H. MD	Inv	1985
Anwar, Khawaja N., MD	Noninv	1982		Klein, Michael MD	Interv	1985
Buafo, Charles K., MD	Noninv	1982		Ramsay, Kenneth, MD	Noninv	1985
Cooper, James C., DO	Inv	1982		Rosenblum, Stephen, MD	Inv	1985
Dickerson, Reginald, MD	Inv	1982		Schaber, Douglas C., DO	Inv	1985
Doyle, Timothy P., MD	Inv	1982		Strobl, David J., DO	Noninv	1985
Esper, William A., DO	Inv	1982		Subich, David C., MD	Noninv	1985
Fugate, Jeffrey S, DO	Inv	1982		Zaidi, Adnan R., MD,	Inv/Interv	1985
Krauthamer, Daniel, MD	Inv	1982		Abi Samra, Freddy M., MD	EP	1986
McGrath, Kenneth G., Jr DO	Inv	1982		Bellamy, Gregory R., MD	Noninv	1986
Murcko, Lawrence G., MD	Inv	1982		Cuddy, Stephen R., MD	Inv	1986
Palaniappan, Jawahar, MD	Noninv	1982		Davis, G. Stefan, MD	Inv/EP	1986
Schen, Sanford E., MD	Noninv	1982		Drummer, Eric M., MD	Inv/Interv	1986
Walborn, A. Mary, MD	Noninv	1982		Furey, Kevin P., DO	Inv/Interv	1986
Williams. Shirley A., MD	Noninv	1982		Ghazi-Zadeh, Freidoon, MD,	Inv	1986
Yiannikas, John, MD	Noninv	1982		Hector, David Alphonso.MD	Inv	1986

Kadri, Nazih, MD	EP	1986
Kaminski, Brian L., MD	Inv	1986
Kreindel, Mark S., MD	Inv	1986
Maglione, Anthony, MD	Noninv	1986
Pollock, Dean M., MD	Inv	1986
Salinger, Michael, MD	Interv	1986
Scheinbach, Alan J., DO	Noninv	1986
Sheehy, Patrick G., MD	Inv	1986
Simmons, Tony, MD	EP	1986
Wilson, John H. MD	Inv	1986
Bear, Phillip A., DO	Inv	1987
Chambers, James L. MD	Inv/Interv	1987
Cooper, Daniel M. MD	EP	1987
Gerber, Elliot M., MD	Inv	1987
Gordon, Terry A, DO,	Inv	1987
Gossman, David, MD	Inv	1987
Kyreakakis, Anthony J.,MD	Inv	1987
McEniery, Paul, MD	Inv/interv	1987
Otero-Cagide, Manuel R., MD	EP	1987
Plavac, Thomas G., MD	Noninv	1987
Prior, Michael I., MD,	Inv/EP	1987
Vacante, Michael, DO	Inv	1987
VanderLaan, Ronald Lee, MD	Inv	1987
Arora, Rohit R., MD	Inv/Interv	1988
Arora, Rohit, MD	Interv	1988
Bournigal, Douglas R., MD	Noninv/Imaging	1988
Divernois, Jaques	Interv	1988
From, Joel MD	Inv	1988
Grigera, Fernando, MD	Inv/Interv	1988
Harrington, J. Frederick, MD	ClinCard	1988
Lenehan, Stephen P., MD	Noninv	1988
Masterson, Martin, MD	EP	1988
Polinski, William J., DO, PhD	Inv	1988
Raymond, Russell E., DO	Inv/Interv	1988
Reed, Mona. MD	Inv	1988
Trono, Ruben, MD	Inv	1988
Vigessa, Gragory MD	Inv	1988
Ballas, Steven, MD	Inv	1989
Brodsky, Marc	Inv	1989
Butler, James R, DO	Inv	1989
Calafiore, Paul, MD	Imaging	1989

Chin, William (Bill) Lang, DO	Noninv	1989
Corbelli, Richard, MD	Inv/EP	1989
Dimas, Alexios P., MD	Inv/Interv Research	1989
Emre, Atila, MD	Research	1989
Horwitz, Edward C., MD	Noninv	1989
Marsalese, Dominic, MD	Inv/Interv	1989
McAlister, Hugh, MD	EP	1989
McCowan, Ronald S., MD	EP	1989
Perona, Philip S., MD	Inv/EP	1989
Platko, William Paul, MD	Inv/Interv	1989
Tuzcu, E. Murat, MD	inv/Interv	1989
Verhey, Margaret H., MD	Inv	1989
Brodell, George K., MD	Inv	1990
Frierson, John, MD	Interv	1990
Harms, Geoffrey L., MD	Inv/Interv	1990
Hughes, Thomas D., DO	Inv	1990
James, Karen, MD	Inv	1990
Marwick, Thomas, MD	Imaging	1990
Obarski, Timothy P., DO	Noninv	1990
Petrella, Richard, MD	Inv/Interv	1990
Pordon, Cynthia, DO	Inv	1990
Rabinowitz, Arthur J., MD,	Inv	1990
Walsh, Timothy, MD	EP	1990
Wunderly, Douglas James, MD	Inv	1990
Abu-Rmalieh, Akef, MD	Noninv	1991
Bartlett, James C., DO	Noninv	1991
Davison, Malcolm MB BS	Imaging	1991
Edel, Thomas, MD	Inv/EP	1991
Font, Vteente E., MD	Noninv	1991
Gohn, Douglas, MD	Inv/EP	1991
Goldman, Martin E.	Noninv	1991
Hazen, Mark, MD	Inv	1991
Hughes, Michael M., MD	Inv/Interv	1991
Mazurek, Robert, MD	Inv	1991
McGuinn, W. Patrick, MD	Inv/EP	1991
Michelson, Barry, MD	Inv	1991
Nemec, James, MD	Noninv	1991
Robalino, Benjamin D., MD	Inv/Interv	1991
Sheares, Reuben A. III, MD	Interv	1991
Sitthisook, Surapun, MD	EP	1991

Vaska, Kevin, MD	Interv	1991	Elliott, John M., MBChB,PhD	Interv	1994
Williams, Deborah, MD	EP	1991	Evans, Daniel J., DO	CARD	1994
Arnold, Anita, MD	InvInterv	1992	Garcia, MarioJ.,MD	Imaging	1994
Barettella, Mark Bernard, MD	Inv	1992	Goodhart, David, MD	CARD	1994
Duffy, Carol, DO	Noninv	1992	Grimm, Richard A., DO	CARD/Imaging	1994
Gulotta, Ronald J., MD	Inv	1992	Hall, Jason O., MD	CARD/Interv	1994
Hagemann, Timothy W., MD	Inv/Interv	1992	Hamer. David, MD	CARD	1994
Hardigan, Kenneth R., MD	Inv	1992	Kleman, James Michael, MD	EP	1994
Horvitz, Lewis, MD	Inv	1992	Lee, Kamthorn, MD	CARD/Imaging	1994
Isada, Loretta R., MD	Noninv	1992	MacIsaac, Andrew MBBS	Interv	1994
Joyce, Frederic S., MD	Inv	1992	McGarvey, Joseph, MD	Noninv	1994
McClure, J. Miles, MD	Inv	1992	Moliterno, David J.,MD	Interv	1994
Mick, Matthew J,MD,	Inv/Interv	1992	Ng, William, MD	CARD	1994
Moore, Stephen L., DO	Inv/EP	1992	Omoigui, Nowa, MD	Interv	1994
Olivares, Gilbert Thomas, MD	Inv	1992	Pacheco, R., MD	CARD	1994
Suri, Rajesh S., MD	EP	1992	Pimentel. Carlos X., MD	CARD	1994
Sutton, Joseph, MD	Interv	1992	Schutzman, Jerome, MD	CARD	1994
Torelli, Julius, MD	Noninv	1992	Alawwa, Abdul, MD	EP	1995
Wendschuh, Philip, MD	Inv	1992	Anderson, Terry, MD	CARD	1995
Abdel Meguid, Alaa E, MD	Interv	1993	Czerska, Barbara, MD	HF	1995
Bernardi, Mark, DO	CARD/Interv	1993	Duerr, Robert L, MD	Interv	1995
Brown, David L, MD	Interv	1993	Eisenberg, Mark J., MD, MPH	Interv	1995
Casale, Paul, MD	CARD	1993	Fahrig, Stephen A., MD	EP	1995
Cliffe, Charles M, II, MD	CARD	1993	Fahy, Gerald, MBBS	EP	1995
Coulis, Louie, MO	CARD	1993	Fritz, Ronald M., DO	CARD	1995
Fix, James S., MD	CARD	1993	Kuhn, Michael, MD	Ped Interv	1995
Jaeger, PredrickJ., DO	CARD/EP	1993	Lefkovits, Jeffrey, MBBS	Interv	1995
Jones, Steven E., MD	CARD/Interv	1993	Miller, Raymond E., MD	Inv/EP	1995
Lincoff, A. Michael, MD	CARD/Interv	1993	Munoz, Fernando X., MD	Inv	1995
McClusky, Edward, MD	Interv	1993	Nakatani, Satoshi, MD, PhD	Imaging	1995
Pietrolungo, Josaeph, MD	CARD	1993	Paranandi, Srinivas N., MD	Inv/Interv	1995
Pinski, Sergio L., MD	EP	1993	Pilote, Louise, MD	CARD/Res	1995
Schutzman, John J., MD	CARD/EP	1993	Pool, Duane P., MD	CARD	1995
Underwood, Paul L., Jr., MD	CARD	1993	Rashid, John Floyd, MD	CARD	1995
Vandervoort, Pieter M.K., MD	CARD	1993	Rodriguez, L. Leonardo, MD	Imaging	1995
Villa, Augusta E., MD	Interv	1993	Schenck, Margaret MD	EP	1995
Weis, Andrew J, MD	Cath/Imaging	1967,1993	Sgarbossa, Ms. Elena B., MD	CARD	1995
Witcik, William, MD	CARD	1993	Weinstock, Martin, MD	EP	1995
Bailey, Joe C., MD	CARD	1994	Almony, Gregory, MD	CARD	1996
Boehrer, James D., MD	Interv	1994	Annan, Kingsley, MD	CARD	1996
DeFranco, Anthony, MD	CARD/Interv	1994	Breburda, Christian, MD	Imaging	1996

Brener, Sorin S., MD	CARD/Interv	1996	Wang, Chao-wen, MD	CARD	1997
Brieger, David, MBBS	Interv	1996	Ward, Samuel, MD	CARD/Interv	1997
Challapalli, Ram, MD	CARD	1996	Williams, M. John, MD	Imaging	1997
Chiu, Andrew Chun-tah, MD,	CARD	1996	Al-Khadra, Ayman S., MD	EP	1998
Coman, James, MD	Inv/EP	1996	Asher, Craig, MD	CARD/Imaging	1998
Dunlap, Stephanie H, DO	HF	1996	Augostini, Ralph Sayre, MD	CARD/EP	1998
Eccleston, David, MD	Interv	1996	Bhalla, H. Bobby, MD	CARD	1998
Gimbel, J. Rod, MD	Inv/EP	1996	Chetcuti, Stanley J.MD	CARD	1998
Gitlin, Jeffrey. MD	Inv/Interv	1996	Erdogan, Okan, MD	EP	1998
Guzman, Luis, MD	CARD/Interv	1996	Farhy, Rodorto 0., MD	CARD	1998
Helguera, Marcello, MD	EP	1996	Grady, Thomas A., MD	CARD	1998
Horrigan, Mark, MD	Interv	1996	Graziano, Joseph A., MD	CARD	1998
Johnson, Todd Lewis, MD	Inv	1996	Gupta, Navin, MD	CARD	1998
Leung, Dominick, MD	Imaging	1996	Kidwell, Gregory A., MD	EP	1998
Li, Steven Siu Lung, MD	Noninv	1996	Kwong, Shu Keung, MD	Noninv	1998
Mak, Koon-Hou, MD	Interv	1996	Main, Michael L, MD	Imaging	1998
Patel, Hiren K., MD	CARD	1996	Mallawi, Yaseen, MD	EP	1998
Ragan, John, MD	CARD	1996	Maragos, Stavros G., MD	CARD	1998
Sheldon, William S., DO	CARD/Interv	1996	Moen, Elaine K., MD	CARD	1998
Weinstock. Martin M., MD	EP	1996	Narins, Craig, MD	Interv	1998
Ballal, Raj Sadananda, MD	CARD	1997	Park, Myung, MD	HF	1998
Belli, Guldo, MD	CARD/Interv	1997	Scott, Robert, MD	HF	1998
Dawson, Irving, MD	CARD/Imaging	1997	Shah, Milind S., MD	CARD	1998
Erickson, Bernard, MD	CARD	1997	Shan, Kesavan, MD	CARD	1998
Foley, Brian. MD	HF	1997	Silver, Mitchell, DO	CARD/Interv/VM	1998
Ghaffari, Sasan, MD	CARD	1997	Steinhubl, Steven R., MD	CARD/Interv	1998
Guetta, Victor, MD	Interv	1997	Wischmeyer, Jason, MD	CARD	1998
Heupler, Stephen MD	CARD	1997	Wong, James, MD	Imaging	1998
Jolly, Neeraj, MD	Interv	1997	Yamada, Elina, MD	Imaging	1998
Lee, Chao-Wen, MD	CARD	1997	Armstrong, Guy P., MD	Imaging	1999
Lee, Karla, MD	CARD	1997	Bajzer, Christopher, MD	CARD/Interv	1999
Mayer Sabik, Ellen Louise, MD	CARD/Imaging	1997	Bowen, Timothy Eric, MD	Cath	1999
Metz, Brian Kevin, MD	CARD	1997	Campbell, Leslie MD	CARD	1999
Migrino, Raymond Q., MD	CARD	1997	Cura, Fernando, MD	Interv	1999
Motwani, Joseph, MD	Interv	1997	Deedy, Matthew,MD	CARD/Interv	1999
Powers, James B., MD	CARD	1997	Ergodan. Okan, MD	EP	1999
Rodkey. Suzanne, MD	CARD/HF	1997	Flachskampf, Frank, MD	Interv	1999
Scalia, Gregory, MD	Imaging	1997	Horner, Simon, MD	Interv	1999
Schloss. Edward, MD	EP	1997	Jaber, Wael, MD	Imaging	1999
Seals. Stevan Eugene, MD	CARD/EP	1997	Marso, Steven, MD	CARD	1999
Tsui, Kin-Lam	Noniniv	1997	Peterson, John G.	CARD	1999

Rabbani, Ramin, MD	CARD/Interv	1999		Lewis, David, MD	CARD	2001
Roe, Matthew	CARD	1999		Mohiuddin, Ishtiaque, MD	Imaging	2001
Rubin, David N., MD	CARD/Imaging	1999		Mukherjee, Debabrata, MD	CARD/Interv	2001
Saliba, Walid I., MD	CARD/EP	1999		Pavia, Steven, MD	EP	2001
Scally, Amy, MD	CARD	1999		Pereirea, Jeremy, MD	Imaging	2001
Shah, Deepak L. MD	CARD	1999		Pu, Min, MD	CARD	2001
Tan, Walter, MD	CARD/Interv	1999		Robbins, Mark, MD	CARD/Interv	2001
Tayara, Wakkas, MD	CARD	1999		Rosario, Adriana, MD	HF	2001
Wahi, Sudhir, MD	Imaging	1999		Yamada, David, MD	CARD	2001
Yamani, M. Hilal, MD	HF	1999		Agah, Ramtin, MD	Interv	2002
Yamanouchi, Yoshio, MD,PhD	RES/EP	1999		Balaban, Krzyszytof, MD	CARD/EP	2002
Albirini. Abdulhay, MD	Interv	2000		Bettadapur, Monica, MD	CARD	2002
Cura, Fernando, MD	Interv	2000		Boyle, Andrew, MD	CARD/HF	2002
deGuise, Michele, MD	HF	2000		Chan, Albert. MD	Interv	2002
Foody, JoAnne, MD	CARD	2000		Cho, Leslie, MD	CARD/Interv	2002
Gassler, John, MD	CARD	2000		Cole, Christopher, MD	CARD/EP	2002
Jimenez, Javier, MD	HF	2000		Colvin, Monica, MD	HF	2002
Kanagaratnam, Logan	EP	2000		Dresing, Thomas, MD	CARD/EP	2002
Kapadia, Samir R, MD	CARD/Interv	2000		Estess, Murray, MD	CARD	2002
L'Allier, Philippe L, MD	CARD/Interv	2000		Gerschutz, Gregory, MD	CARD	2002
Lauer, Michael, MD	CARD/Interv	2000		Hayek, Emil, MD	CARD	2002
Lin, Steve Sheng-Hsiu, MD	CARD/Imaging	2000		Khot, Umesh, MD	CARD	2002
Murphy, Mark T., MD	CARD/Imaging	2000		Mahon, Niall, MD	HF	2002
Nadar, Simon, MD	CARD/HF	2000		Masri, Kalil, MD	HF	2002
Patel, Vasant, MD	CARD	2000		Monson, Michael, MD	CARD	2002
Penn, Marc S., MD	CARD	2000		Novaro, Gian, MD	CARD/Imaging	2002
Prior, David, MD	Imaging	2000		Obenza-Nishime, Erna, MD	CARD/HF	2002
Saligan, Josephine, MD	CARD/EP	2000		Quinn, Martin, MD	Interv	2002
Saligan, Josephine, MD	EP	2000		Roffi, Marco, MD	Interv	2001
Schweikert, Robert, MD	CARD/EP	2000		Smith, Rebecca, MD	Imaging	2002
Skiles, Jeffrey Alien. MD	CARD	2000		Vlassak, Irmien, MD	Imaging	2002
Smith, John Horatio, II, MD	CARD	2000		Yu, David, MD	CARD	2002
Tayara, Wakkas, MD	CARD/HF	2000		Aronow, Herbert, MD	CARD/Interv	2003
Thamilarasan, Maran, MD	CARD/Imaging	2000		Askari, Arman, MD	CARD	2003
Wu. Jenny, MD	CARD	2000		Aviles, Ron, MD	CARD	2003
Ziada, Khaled. MD	Interv	2000		Dauterman, Kent, MD	Interv	2003
Abreu, Miquel, MD	EP	2001		Ellis, Keith, MD	CARD	2003
Bhatt, Deepak L, MD	CARD/Interv	2001		Gum, Particia, MD	CARD/Interv	2003
Chew, Derek, MD	Interv	2001		Marrouche, Nassir, MD	EP	2003
Diaz, Lazaro, MD	CARD	2001		McRae, Tom, MD	CARD/HF	2003
Lam, Cathy, MD	EP	2001		Merritt, Chris, MD	CARD	2003

183

Messerli, Adrian, MD	CARD	2003		Civello, Kenneth, MD	CARD	2005
Ng, Kenneth, MD	Imaging	2003		Cotroneo, John, MD	Imaging	2005
Reginelli, Joel, MD	CARD/Interv	2003		Cummings, Jennifer, MD	EP	2005
Saad, Eduardo, MD	EP	2003		Dubois, Nicholas, MD	CARD HF	2005
Salazar, Holger, MD	Imaging	2003		Fathi, Robert, MD	Interv	2005
Schoenhagen, Paul, MD	CARD/CT-MRI	2003		Fitzgerald, Ben, MD	Imaging	2005
Seshadri, Niranjan, MD	CARD	2003		Grant, Celeste Thomas, MD	HF	2005
Tamberella, Michael, MD	CARD	2003		Gring, Christian, MD	CARD HF	2005
Troughton, Richard, MD	Imaging/HF	2003		Gurm, Hitinder, MD	CARD/Interv	2005
Abdul-Karim, Ahmad, MD	EP	2004		Hesse, Barbara, MD	CARD/Imaging	2005
Atkeson, Benjamin, MD	CARD	2004		Hook, Matthew, MD	CARD/Interv	2005
Burkhardt, John, MD	EP	2004		Jefferson, Brian, MD	CARD/HF	2005
Casserly, Ivan, MD	CARD/Interv	2004		Joseph, George, MD	EP	2004
Exaire, Emilio, MD	Interv	2004		Kalahasti, Sagar, MD	CARD/HF	2005
Haery, Cameron. MD	Interv	2004		Khan, Mohammed, MD	CARD/HF	2005
Hostetter, Jack, MD	CARD	2004		Lakkireddy, Dhanunjaya, MD	EP	2005
Huang, Julie, MD	CARD	2004		Lalude, Omosalewa, MD	Imaging	2005
Jones, Chris, MD	CARD	2004		Lee, David, MD	CARD/Interv	2005
Khaykin, Yaariv, MD	EP	2004		Maroo, Anjli, MD	CARD/Interv	2005
Nash, Patrick, MD	Imaging/HF	2004		McWilliams, Michael, MD	CARD	2005
O'Neill, James, MD	HF	2004		Murphy, Ross, MD	HF, Imaging	2006
Sachar, Ravish, MD	CARD/Interv	2004		Ozduran, Volkan, MD	HF	2005
Sallach, John, MD	Imaging	2004		Rajagopal, Vivek, MD	CARD	2005
Saw, Jacqueline, MD	Interv	2004		Sauri, Daniel, MD	CARD	2005
Sigurdsson, Gardar, MD	Imaging	2004		Simpfendorfer, Christian, MD	CARD	2005
Sleik, Khaled, MD	Imaging	2004		Verma, Atul, MD	EP	2005
Srichai, Barbara, MD	CARD/Imaging	2004		Vivekananthan, Deepak, MD	CARD/Interv	2005
Stehlik, Josef, MD	HF	2004		Wazni, Oussama, MD	CARD/EP	2005
Tang, Wilson, MD	CARD/HF	2004		William, Timothy, MD	HF	2005
Tschopp, David, MD	CARD	2004		Yen, Michael, MD	CARD/Interv	2005
Xu, Xiao Fang, MD	Imaging	2003				
Ziada, Khaled, MD	CARD	2004				
Zidar, Frank, MD	CARD	2004				
Bailey, Shane, MD	CARD	2005				
Barman, Nitin, MD	CARD	2005				
Belden, William, MD	EP	2005				
Bhargava, Mandeep, MD	EP	2005				
Chacko, Matthew, MD	CARD	2005				
Chen, Michael, MD	CARD/Interv	2005				
Chiu, John, MD	CARD/Interv	2005				
Chuang, Hsuan-Hung, MD	HF	2005				

CARD = general cardiology including noninvasive and diagnostic catheterization
Cath (later Inv) = cardiology including diagnostic cardiac catheterization
ClinCard = clinical cardiology
CT-MRI = computerized tomographic and magnetic resonance cardiac imaging
EP = pacemakers and electrophysiology
HF = heart failure
IM = internal medicine
Interv = interventional cardiology
Noninv = clinical cardiology

VM = vascular medicine

APPENDIX 3

CARDIOLOGY LEADERSHIP POSITIONS

		Department of Cardiorespiratory Disease/Cardiovascular Disease/Clinical Cardiology				
	ERNSTENE 1932-1965					
		Department of Clinical Cardiology PROUDFIT 1965-1974				
		Department of Pediatric Cardiol/ CV Disease/ Cardiac Labratory SONES 1960-1975				
			Department of Cardiology SHELDON 1975-1991			
Sections						
Clinical Cardiology			Lewis 1975-1992			
Cath Lab Clinical Section			Shirey 1975-1989	Heupler 1989-1991		
ECG	Proudfit 1946-1966	Westcott 1966-1973	Lewis 1973-1986	Underwood 1986-		
Cardiac Function Laboratory		Siegel 1971-1977	Salcedo 1977-1992			
Nuclear Cardiology			Salcedo/Rincon/Cook 1977-			
CHIRP Cardiac Rehabilitation			Underwood/Blackburn 1985-1989		Pashkow/Blackburn 1989-	
Pacemakers/EPS		Castle 1973-	Castle 1973-1994			
EPS Laboratories			Maloney 1981-1992			
Ambulatory Electrocardiography (Holter, Telemetry)			Morant 1982-			
Sones Cath Labs			Shirey 1975-1988	Heupler 1989-1991		
Interventional			Phillips 1982-1983	Hollman 1983-1990	Whitlow 1990-	
Pediatric Cardiology			Moodie 1978-1987	Sterba 1987		
Heart Failure-Transplantation						
Coronary Intensive Care		Lewis 1970-1973	Hodgman 1973-1986	Whitlow 1986-1988	Jubran 1988-1992	
Committees						

185

Education			Razavi 1975-1979	Heupler/Hart 1979-1982	Heupler/ Salcedo 1982-1985	Hobbs/ Underwood 1985-1991	
Medical Students			Hart 1975-1980	Underwood 1980-2004			
Internal Medicine Rotators			Hobbs 1984-1991				
Departmental Assistants			Phillips 1978-1979	Phillips/ Hodgman 1979-1981	Hodgman 1981-1985	Hodgman/ Dorosti 1985-1990	Hodgman 1990-1991
Research			Proudfit 1975-1980	Salcedo 1980-1986	Stewart 1986-1991		
Patient Care			Hodgman/ Phillips 1982-1983	Hodgman-Razavi 1983-1991			
Appointment Desk Advisory		Lim 1975-1990	Morant 1990-1998				
Computer Applications Task Force	Moodie 1984-1986	Sheldon 1987-1989	Wilkoff 1989-				
Administrative Director		Florio 1974-1987	Petrovlc 1985-				

186

Appendix 3 (Cont) Cardiology Leadership Positions

TOPOL 1991-2006					
Vice Chairman		Nissen 1993-2002	Young 2002-2003	Griffin 2003-	
Sections					
Clinical Cardiology	Underwood 1991;	Nissen 1992-1999	Rimmerman 1999-2004	Francis 2004-	
Cath Lab Clinical Section	Ellis 1991				
ECG	Underwood 1986-				
ECG Core Laboratory		Underwood 1997-			
Cardiac Function Laboratory	*Imaging* Salcedo 1977-92	Thomas 1992-			
Nuclear Cardiology					
CHIRP Cardiac Rehabilitation	Pashkow/Blackburn 1989-				
Echocardiograph Laboratory		Stewart 1993-			
Imaging Research		Klein 1993-			
Valve Management Center		Griffin 1993-			
Intravascular Ultrasound Laboratory		Nissen 1994-			
Pacemakers/EPS	*Electrophysiology* Castle 1973-1994	Tchou 1994-	Co-directors Tchou and Natale 2001-2005	Natale 2005-2007	
EPS Laboratories		Kidwell 1996-1998			
Ambulatory Electrocardiography (Holter, Telemetry)	Morant 1992-1998	Jaeger 1998-			
Atrial Fibrillation Clinic		Chung 1995-			
Implantable Device Clinic		Wilkoff 1996-			
Sones Cath Labs	*Invasive* Ellis 1991-				
Interventional	*Interventional* Whitlow 1990-1992				
Vascular Interventions			Yadav 2001-2006		
Experimental Interventional Laboratory		Lincoff 1993-			
Pediatric Cardiology	*Congenital* Sterba 1987-1993	Latson 1993-1994			
Heart Failure-Transplantation	Hobbs 1991-1995	Young 1995-2003	Starling 2003-		
Clinical Trial Director		Hobbs 1995-			
HTx Services Director		Starling 1995-			
Dir Sp Care Unit		Haas 1995-2000			
Kaufman Center for Heart Failure			1997- McCarthy—Surgical Young—Medical		
Vascular Medicine			Ruschaupt 2001-2002	Linda Graham 2002-2004	Bartholomew 2004-

187

Vascular Laboratory			LaPerna 2001-		
Peripheral Intervention Lab			Yadav 2001-2006		
Coronary Intensive Care	Jubran 1988-1992	Nissen 1992-1997	Francis 1997- Co-Director Lauer		
Preventive Cardiology		Sprecher 1995-2003	Stanley Hazen 2003-		
Consult Service	Pashkow 1991-				
Surgical Service		1992-			
Committees					
Education	Hobbs/Salcedo 1991-	Black 1992-1994	Griffin 1994-		
Ernstene, Shirey Teaching Services		Underwood 1993-1997	Rimmerman 1997-		
Medical Students				Stewart 2004-	
Internal Medicine Rotators					
Departmental Assistants					
Research					
Patient Care					
Appointment Desk Advisory					
Computer Applications Task Force	Wilkoff 1989-1996	Lauer 1996-			
Angiographic Core Laboratory	Ellis/ Dobowey 1991-1998		Ivanc 1998-		
Intravascular Ultrasound Core Laboratory	Nissen 1993-1995	Nissen/Tuzcu 1995-1998	Tuzcu /Crowe 1998-		
Graphics and Design	Dobowey 1991-1998		Moss 1998-		
Center for Thrombosis and Vascular Biology		Plow 1993-			
Clinical Trials Unit	Stosic 1991-1995	Incl Interventional Registry 1994- C5 Cleveland Clinic Cardiovascular Coordinating Unit 1995-	DeLuca 1995-		
Administrative Director	Petrovic 1985-				

www.ingramcontent.com/pod-product-compliance
Lightning Source LLC
Chambersburg PA
CBHW032003170526
45157CB00002B/524